CW01656725

Youniform

Youniform

A Revolutionary Style System to Simplify Your Wardrobe for Good

STACEY HERNDON

Joyful Talents Press

Youniform: The Revolutionary Style System to Simplify Your Wardrobe for Good
Copyright © 2026 by Stacey Herndon

Published in the United States by Joyful Talents Press, an imprint of Joyful Talents LLC, Texas. All rights reserved. No part of this publication may be reproduced, distributed, or transmitted in any form or by any means, including photocopying, recording, or other electronic or mechanical methods, without the prior written permission of the publisher, except in the case of brief quotations embodied in critical reviews and certain other noncommercial uses permitted by copyright law.

Some images in this book are used under Creative Commons licenses. Brand images are used under fair use doctrine. Unless otherwise noted, all other images, graphics, and visual materials are the intellectual property of Stacey Herndon and/or her affiliated companies, including Marvelous Works LLC and Joyful Talents LLC. Radiantly Dressed®, Radiant Woman®, Youniform™, Youniform Framework™, Five Stages of Style™, Color Coded Closet™, Style Goals™, You Essentials™, 4-Piece Wardrobe™, 7 Foolproof Outfits™, Big Four Seasons™, Essence Map™, ColorEssence™, Get Dressed. Be Radiant.™, and Radiant Life™ are trademarks of Stacey Herndon, Marvelous Works LLC, and Joyful Talents LLC.

This book is intended for educational and informational purposes only. It reflects the author's experience and professional work in personal style and image consulting. While it addresses confidence and self-image as they relate to personal style, it is not intended to diagnose, treat, or replace professional medical, psychological, or therapeutic care. The information and methods described in this book do not constitute a guarantee of results. Personal style is inherently individual, and outcomes may vary based on personal preferences, circumstances, and application. The author assumes no responsibility or liability for how the information in this book is used.

The stories, examples, and case studies shared in this book are drawn from real client experiences. Names and identifying details have been changed to protect privacy. Any resemblance to actual persons, living or deceased, outside of these real client relationships is purely coincidental. Websites, links, and online resources referenced in this book were accurate at the time of publication. Due to the dynamic nature of the internet, some links may change or become unavailable over time.

Library of Congress Control Number: 2026903053

ISBN: 979-8-9941542-2-9 (paperback)
ISBN: 979-8-9941542-1-2 (e-book)
ISBN: 979-8-9941542-3-6 (hardcover)
ISBN: 979-8-9941542-4-3 (audiobook)

For the thousands of women I have had the privilege to serve.

Thank you for trusting me with your stories and inviting me into your lives. May your clothes always be the outward expression of a life fully surrendered to what matters most.

Contents

To the Reader XI

Acknowledgements XIII

Introduction XV

Part One: Why Getting Dressed Feels so Hard

1. The Chaotic Morning 3
    - Your Brain Needs You to Stop Overthinking...
    - Do You Have Enough Willpower?
    - How to Dress Like the Woman You're Becoming
2. The Perfect Closet 19
    - When Clothing Stopped Being Valuable
    - The Human Cost of Modern Fashion
    - Why Expensive Doesn't Mean Quality
    - How to Buy Clothes that Last
    - Clothes Don't Die Quietly
3. Just One Dress 43
    - No One Notices What You're Wearing (Seriously)
    - How Comparison Culture Hijacked Personal Style
    - What Fashion Reveals About Our Need to Belong
    - The Real Reason You Wear the Same Things

Why Most Women Never Claim Their Style

Part Two: The Youniform System

4. The Five Stages of Style 65
   The Cool Closet Reset that Builds Your Confidence
   Create Clarity in 30 Minutes with the Style Goals Exercise
   This Exercise Will Transform How You See Your Body Forever
   Design Your Closet with Intention and Get Dressed in Five Minutes Flat
   The Secret to Staying Effortlessly Stylish for Life

5. One Great Outfit 97
   The Real Reason Successful People Repeat Outfits
   You Need More Than a Black Tee and Jeans
   How to Create Variety in a Style Youniform
   One Youniform = 384 Days of Style

6. 7 Outfits for Life 117
   What No One Tells You About Capsule Wardrobes
   The Style System Hidden in Your Routine
   Create the Perfect Youniform for Every Moment
   The Only Seven Outfits You'll Ever Need
   Master Mix-and-Match Style with Zero Guesswork
   Style Icons Who Rely on Signature Youniforms

Part Three: Personal Style, Applied to You

7. The Biggest Style Breakthrough 147
   The First Style Win Every Woman Needs

How to Identify Your Color Season With Confidence
Build Your Wardrobe With Just 11 Colors

8. Embrace the Real You 167
The Message You're Sending Without Saying a Word
How to Find Your Unique Style Through Essence Mapping
Creating the Perfect Style for Every Moment

9. Natural Bodies 185
What Traditional Body Typing Never Told You
This One Thing is the Key to Dressing Your Body
How to Accentuate the Body You Actually Have
Make Friends with the Woman in the Mirror

10. The Stylish Woman 213
The Power of a Master Shopping List
Holding On is Holding You Back
Style Is Not Meant to Stay the Same
How to Actually Get Dressed in Two Minutes

11. Get Dressed. Be Radiant. 235
Your Morning Sets the Tone for Your Whole Day
Make Great Style Part of Your Legacy
Becoming a Radiant Woman

Appendix A: ColorEssence Seasons 249
System Overview
ColorEssence Spring Seasons
ColorEssence Summer Seasons

ColorEssence Autumn Seasons
ColorEssence Winter Seasons
Appendix B: Youniform Activities 273
Recommended Reading 279
References 281
About the Author 289
Let's Connect 291

To the Reader

I started dreaming of this book in 2023, but I wasn't ready to write it. Knowing what I know now, I definitely didn't have the right headspace to bring a book into the world. And even though I've dreamed of being an author for decades, I never imagined that my debut would be this topic.

But personal style is the business I built and everyone says its a good fit. My brain loves to pick things apart, find the golden nuggets, and put them back together in ways that make sense. I like to think of it as efficiently moving forward. How-to information is my bread and butter, and you will get a firehose in this book.

Which brings me to the first warning...I don't do shallow. We joke behind the scenes of the business that I struggle to edit. Our programs tend to get bigger than planned because I go deep into topics. This was great when writing a book, because there was an endless amount of helpful content.

But the reason I didn't know how to get started those years ago, was that I didn't know how to make it all flow. I had heard of the Hero's Journey for storytelling, and knew I wanted to weave it into the teaching content. But I didn't know how until I met my amazing book coach.

This is the second warning...there are lots of stories. Mine and my clients. One of my beta readers mentioned that she wanted to rush through them to get to the meat, but I would encourage you to enjoy them as they come.

Our lives are a tapestry of the experiences we've had, and personal style is a direct outcome. My perspectives and the things I'm teaching you come from those little moments that pop up.

The final warning is that you must do the work. There are over thirty activities in this book to help you explore style, and even more introspection moments.

Take them.

Use them to dress well and live even better.

Thank you for joining me on the adventure of personal style.

YOUNIFORMBOOK.COM

Acknowledgements

To my husband, *Joshua*—thank you for always supporting my ideas and brainstorms. For being my person in this crazy big life with all these humans we made. "Just wait five years..."

To my beautiful children (*who shall remain unnamed for their privacy*)—thank you for giving me a reason to wake up every day and try to be a better person. For showing me the infinite uniqueness in every soul, and that love multiplies exponentially.

To my book coach extraordinaire *Holly*—thank you for creating a book development system that makes my organized brain happy. For every Telegram meltdown and providing a consistent encouraging presence for the whole journey.

To my assistant *Emily*—thank for you embracing the mission and keeping the wheels turning when I am working on projects. For encouraging and embracing our clients to be the very best versions of themselves.

To my assistant *LaToya*—thank you for always being up for trying something new and putting into place my endless experiments in this vast online space.

To my Beta readers, *Mary, Melinda, Annie*—thank you for embracing the philosophy of Youniform and for your attention to detail to get this book ready to publish.

To my original encouragers, *Becki, Danielle, and Alessandra*—thank you for taking a chance and jumping in with both feet when I first started.

To my business coach, *Jen*—thank for you the mindset pushes to focus on the big things, instead of getting stuck in the little things.

To my first mentor, *Jamie*—thank you for taking a chance on me and helping me see the value in writing a book. You are a true gem.

To my *parents*—thank you for always being a safe place to land and giving me a complex and rich heritage to build my life.

To *God*—thank you for the gifts and strengths that allow me to impact the lives of others, for the dreams to build a legacy, and for grace undeserved.

Introduction

This isn't a book about fashion. It's a book about living on purpose, and getting dressed with legacy in mind. I'm not going to show you how to be stylish for the sake of being stylish. I'm going to ask you to dream about your life, then build a wardrobe that you can leverage to accomplish big things. I'm going to challenge you to live in full alignment with who you are on the inside, and how you look on the outside. But I'm also going to show you a foolproof way to create beautiful, stunning, repeatable outfits for every single part of your life.

I see you, walking into your closet every day, frustrated and overwhelmed when you try to create an outfit from all the choices hanging in your closet.

You're probably saving it for the last minute, walking in feeling a bit stressed at putting some clothes together. You begin with a positive attitude and choose a top and bottom for your outfit. But it's not right, so you take it off and toss it to the side, not even taking the time to put it away properly.

The process repeats with outfit idea number two, but that one is also a miss, so you add it to the pile. You glance at the clock...five minutes left until you have to be ready to leave. You go for outfit number three–the hail Mary–because let's face it, you don't have time to try again.

This is the outfit you're wearing today, whether you really like it or not (you probably don't, to be honest). But you've run out of time, and to add insult to injury, you have a *discarded pile of frustration* to deal with later.

But maybe there's another option—that you don't even try at all. You default to something easy and "safe"...maybe old leggings and a sweatshirt, or jeans and a faded tee. You're sure there's some secret that other women know about how to be stylish, but since you missed it, you've just given up.

The method I'm about to share with you flips everything the fashion industry has taught you about getting dressed. They would have you believe that you must wander aimlessly through stores, choosing items based on impulse or dopamine. But truly stylish women know the secret I'm about to share: the power of creating style Youniforms. And by the end of this book, you'll know exactly how to be one of them in clothes that show the world your inner beauty.

The only reason I know all this is because of the journey that started when the whole internet said I couldn't create a capsule wardrobe without separates. But I desperately wanted a capsule of just dresses, and in the process of figuring it out, I realized I had the answer all along. It was hidden in a way of dressing I had been subconsciously practicing my entire adult life, modeled to me in childhood. The framework just needed a name and process that could help others. I didn't expect that finding my personal style and simplifying my closet would open doors I only dreamed about. What started as my frustration building a capsule wardrobe turned into a movement that has helped over 2,700 women simplify their style and step into their best life.

For too many years I was that second woman defaulting to wearing *whatever* because I didn't care how I looked. My sense of style disappeared when I became a mom, and the supportive squeeze of maternity pants was my permanent friend postpartum. (I even tried to convince my mom they were the perfect pants). I lived in saggy bottom jeans and maternity tops for a good three years before going down the print leggings fad which shall not be named. Motherhood was beautiful, but I didn't feel that way anymore, and I felt like a stranger in my own body.

But one day I decided I was tired of feeling like a hot mess mom. For months I had been playing a virtual fashion game on my phone, complete with contests and team challenges. I was the leader of the team and spent real money buying digital clothes and hairstyles. After being at homeschool co-op one day and admiring another mom's puffer vest, it hit me...if I cared enough about fashion to pour my time and real money into a game, maybe it was time to invest in my real-world style. That was the day I deleted the game and decided that my motherhood was worth more than hand me down maternity clothes and cheap leggings.

My editor wants me to tell you about all the doors it opened, but the meaning it created is in the mundane moments of my life. My marriage got better because I started to become more authentic. I was a better mom because I had the space to face old demons and start to break negative cycles. And I had the voice to share my experiences and encourage other women to be bold and unashamed of who they really are. Recently, it opened the door to write this book so I could share that same message with you.

By the end of this book you'll have a full understanding of the process of style transformation, from uncovering the style you were born with, to organizing your closet and outfits in a way that truly successful people use. But more than tactics, you will be a different woman: confident, complemented, beautiful, powerful, purposeful, and transformed.

Personal style is both an internal and external expression, and we will explore both sides. In the first chapter, we'll uncover why mornings feel so hard, and how you can get dressed in five minutes to make them easier. In chapter two, you'll find out exactly why those cute outfits you see on other people don't work for you. In chapter three I'll share the low point of my style journey, and maybe you'll see yourself in my mistakes.

As we move into creating Youniforms, you'll discover in chapter four the circular process of style and discover where to start. In chapter five you'll realize that you already have great style, and what you need to do to expand it. Chapter six is for the rest of your life; from sick days to sexy dates, you'll see how the Youniform Framework covers it all. Most women end up with more than one Youniform, because daily life happens in multiple contexts. This chapter will show you how those additional Youniforms work together to support your entire week.

The final chapters explore advanced style tactics to help you look your best. In chapter seven I'll share the single concept that makes your style 50% better. Chapter eight introduces the mental shift that you were born with great style (and shows you how to find it). In chapter nine you'll find out why I hate the traditional body shape theory and what to do instead. And since nothing stays the same for long, chapter ten covers wardrobe maintenance tips for shopping and decluttering. In the final chapter you take control of your own Youniform journey and explore how your life will change when you simplify your style.

After you've completed the steps in this book, you'll have a modular Youniform wardrobe that makes getting dressed every day easy, and a closet filled with clothes you are excited to wear. But you'll also be a woman who gets dressed on purpose, so that you can launch yourself into each day to experience every moment fully present, advancing your life's calling and legacy with each meaningful second.

But first we have to start where it all begins, with you standing in front of your closet each day, wasting time and energy choosing what to wear. We must break your morning cycle before we can build your Youniform closet.

Part One

Why Getting Dressed Feels So Hard

"One of the things I was struggling with was just the sheer number of options which seemed overwhelming. I longed for the simplicity I saw in my husband's closet. I didn't want to wear menswear but just the recipe: button up shirt, trousers, black or brown belt to match his black or brown shoes, if fancier add a tie and suit jacket, if casual sub in jeans and shorter sleeves and possibly sneakers.

"But women's clothing felt like there's so much variety and so many things that don't work together. But now that I have a Youniform, I have that recipe tailored to me and my body and my lifestyle. I lean a bit more formal so my go-to Youniform looks like: fitted trousers, blouse, sweater/cardigan, flats, matching purse/bag (+belt if desired), and accessories. Stacey's system helped me to better edit my closet so the items I kept were in colours and silhouettes and styles that suited me making mixing and matching a lot less struggle. Instead of feeling overwhelmed and stressed by my closet, opening it up feels easy and enjoyable again."

Hilary

One

The Chaotic Morning

"A good decision is based on knowledge and not on numbers." – Plato

Why do we get dressed? We could argue that it is required as part of modern society to cover our private bits. But the nuances of personal style mean we choose clothes for a variety of convoluted reasons. The most compelling purpose is the presentation of some truth about ourselves to the outside world. Often in our desire to be accepted, we forget who we truly are. And as we struggle to fit ourselves into the mold of someone else's life, we lose sight of the things that matter most to us. Our closets get bloated with pretty, shiny things that don't actually suit our lives. Then we steal time from the people who matter most, obsessing over what to wear.

The average woman owns over 100 pieces of clothing. Various studies show that number to be anywhere from 103 to over 200, but this might be a significant underestimate, since people with extensive wardrobes may not want to take surveys (WRAP 2013). When that number is further broken down, the findings become more alarming:

- 21% of a woman's wardrobe is unwearable (damaged, stained, dirty, misplaced, etc.)
- 33% is too tight or small
- 24% is too loose or large
- 12% is unworn/ignored

This leaves approximately 10% of your wardrobe in use at any given time. When you consider the 21% that might be usable but unavailable, the statistics of clothing flow into the Pareto Principle. This states that 20% of effort makes up 80% of output. In clothing terms, you wear 20% of your clothing 80% of the time. Even if you never did the math, you know this to be true. How often have you felt frustrated because your favorite jeans were dirty and the other options were inferior?

Which begs the question: If we're only wearing about 20% of what we own, why does getting dressed feel so hard? Klerk (2016) found that the average woman spends 17 minutes a day choosing what to wear.

That's over 100 hours every single year, which is four entire days lost to the process of getting dressed.

I don't know about you, but the thought of losing four days a year depresses me. Life is just too precious to waste even a single hour. For high-capacity women with big goals, 100 hours can be life-changing. Imagine this: you're on an amazing Alaskan cruise, with a perfect assortment of clothes packed, waking up to a stunning snowy mountain view while sipping coffee with your family on the balcony. Or picture yourself finally launching that passion project you've been putting off for years because you never had the time, and the excitement you feel at your first client. Instead of spending your life reacting to your surroundings, you have the time and intention to pursue actions and choices that create lasting memories.

Every day we make hundreds of decisions, and most of them are insignificant. It seems counterintuitive right now to suggest that the clothes we choose are one of those, but ultimately it is minor in relation to all of the other decisions we make. We often overemphasize minor decisions and deemphasize more important ones. Regardless of what we choose, we possess finite processing power to use each day.

Decision fatigue is a phrase used to explain how our brains become exhausted with each consecutive decision we make. It's a psychological phenomenon that refers to the declining quality of the decisions we make after a long session of decision-making. In other words, the more choices we have to make, the worse we get at making them. It's a daily struggle that affects everyone—from CEOs to homemakers—and it plays a significant role in your daily wardrobe choices as well.

From the moment you wake, you face choices. When the alarm goes off, will you hit the snooze button or get up immediately? Will you stretch to wake up your joints, or will you skip it? You walk to the bathroom with phone in hand; which app will you open first? In the kitchen, you face your first healthy choice: will it be water first or coffee?

You know it's best to get dressed before the kids, so it's time to get yourself ready. Can you use dry shampoo for one more day or will you choose a shower and clean hair? Clarifying shampoo or moisturizing? Straight hair or curly? What color lipstick will you apply? When you start putting on clothes, the decisions suddenly increase exponentially. Pants, shirt, blazer/cardigan, shoes, earrings, necklace—that's six choices if you get them right on the first try.

For those keeping count, we're up to fourteen decisions right now, and that's before you've had breakfast or gotten your kids ready for the day. You still have to wake up your kids and help them make decisions: getting up the easy way or the hard way, what they will wear, did everyone brush their teeth, which shoes are good for the weather. Then breakfast comes, and if you didn't plan ahead, you must choose on the fly based on how much time you have left, your energy level, and how picky your kids are. Finally, you're almost out the door, but those last-minute questions come up: Did you get the permission slip? Do you have your project? Where is your briefcase? and so on. Each moment that you have to stop, think, and consider is a micro-decision.

By the time you leave the house every morning, it is estimated that you've made 30-40 decisions. That's in just a few short hours, in the comfort of your own home, simply getting ready for the day ahead. It's staggering to think about how many decisions you make during the other 14-ish hours of awake time. Thank goodness for sleep!

When we look back at the decisions made during the morning frenzy, we need to consider how we can reduce the number. Automating processes is one of the best ways to reduce unnecessary decision-making. In the above example, there are several ways this can be done, from scheduling shower days, to creating a breakfast meal plan, or preparing your kids' clothes the night before, and systemizing your own closet.

Recently I spoke at a summit, and as I shared about decision fatigue with the host, she suddenly stopped me and said,

"Were you in my room this morning? Because this is me every day. I tried on three different outfits before landing on this shirt," as she gestured to a simple black tee.

A week later, Dana messaged me privately to say she had implemented a style Youniform. She was so eager to tell me her multiple outfit routine had ended. She can finally get dressed in five minutes, and said her husband noticed she was less frazzled in the mornings.

Whatever your situation, imagine your own life and the way you handle your mornings. Some of you have older children and work outside the home. Some of you may have more flexible days where you aren't required to leave the house by a certain time. Maybe you don't have children, allowing more time for personal development and exercise. Regardless of your lifestyle, I challenge you to list out the decisions you make every day. Use your phone and the voice memo function to record what you do on a typical morning. Upload it to an AI-powered analysis app and ask it to analyze your mornings and suggest ways to streamline your decisions. Are you surprised by how much your brain is working in the tiny details? Did you identify a few places where it's time to create systems?

Your Brain Needs You to Stop Overthinking...

Now that you know that decision fatigue is a real thing that affects everyone, it's easy to brush it aside with the excuse that no one is immune. But we are responsible for our own lives and managing the intricacies. Decision fatigue is more than an annoyance or a tally of micro choices we make each day. Making decisions starts a cascade of physical and psychological processes with which our entire body must now contend.

Decision-making takes brainpower, and our brains are sugar monsters. Every cell in our body uses glucose for energy, and the higher functions of the brain demand approximately half of all the glucose in our body (Edwards 2016). This is why experts tell you to eat a balanced breakfast full of healthy carbs, since your brain needs fuel. If one of my kids struggles during a homeschool lesson, I'll often tell them to "go eat a snack because your brain needs glucose."

Your brain is working whether or not you fuel it, which is why we need all the help we can get with deciding what to wear.

In the field of neuroscience, decision making is a fascinating study, because it requires many processes and uses different parts of the brain (Dabir 2024). When we make a decision, we must first evaluate all the options, then we move into consideration and weigh the options, before finally landing on a course of action. Within the structure of the brain, various interactions occur during this process. The prefrontal cortex is the executive center and helps us make decisions based on past experiences and future goals. The limbic system controls many of our feelings, and processes emotions and memories to help us make choices. Neurotransmitters like dopamine and serotonin play a role in our mood and reward pathways about how we choose to move forward.

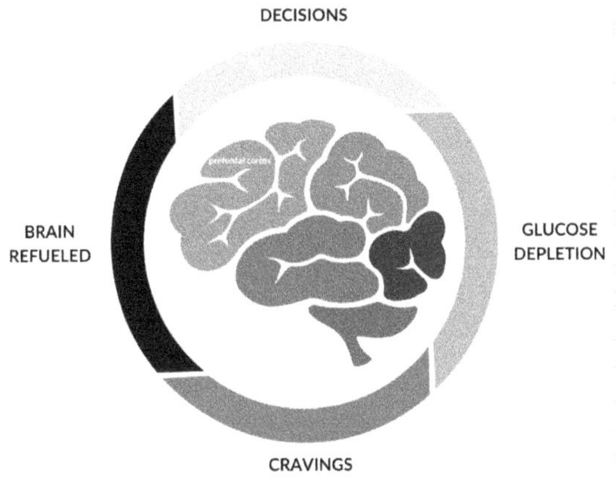

Figure 1.1 Glucose driven decision making occurs in the prefrontal cortex in the brain (for full color images visit youniformbook.com)

Our big "sugar monster" brain is like a computer managing a million tasks to keep us alive and functioning at a high level. Imagine your computer crashing from too many tabs—that's what happens to us when we have too many decisions to make. Everything just crashes and stops working. When we consider the brain as a finite taskmaster, the trickle-down effects of making unnecessary decisions influence the rest of our lives.

Often, our decisions require critical analysis, but when our brain is exhausted from 30+ choices before we leave the house, we cannot see all the potential downfalls. As our brains become overwhelmed with dozens of inconsequential decisions, we become paralyzed and think *every* decision is important, marking an inability to prioritize. If you've ever felt frozen instead of moving forward, it's a clear sign that your decision-making abilities are maxed.

You're making too many decisions, half of which are meaningless.

The opposite of freezing is making decisions on impulse, like when you're standing in the checkout line at the grocery store feeling tired and hungry, and you grab a Mountain Dew at 7 p.m., knowing it will keep you up for hours. Your momentary weakness brings on frustration with yourself, negative self-talk about your character, and crankiness that spills into your relationships. This is why so many women who have big, glorious dreams feel like they're tapped out constantly, overwhelmed and never accomplishing all they know they're meant to do.

You're making too many decisions, half of which are meaningless. "All of this," you ask, "just from choosing what to wear?"

Yes, and no. Yes, because most women linger and agonize over this decision. No, because it's not as important as we make it, and it can be automated. As each of your busy, meaningful days winds down, how do you feel? Are you calm and ready to unwind and sleep? Or do you find yourself frantic and overwhelmed, unable to make one more decision, overstimulated and frozen, just surviving until the day is over? Reducing decision making about what to wear is something that impacts everyone and is just one powerful shift we can hone to conserve our brainpower for bigger things.

Do You Have Enough Willpower?

Some days I wake up with the energy to take on the world, and I accomplish a dozen things and feel like a superhero. On other days, I get dragged out of bed by kids, stumble to my recliner, drink too many cups of coffee, and end the day painfully exhausted with my house looking like a tornado swept through. For many of us, our willpower and energy fluctuate from day to day; even simple things like hormones can play a big role.

This is where the idea of "spoon theory" has always resonated with me.

In my house, we have a problem keeping spoons. One day I'll realize we have one left, then I'll buy a ton of inexpensive spoons because they're obviously being lost or thrown away by small children. Then everyone complains that the silverware drawer barely closes because we have too many. It's a funny story, but we can use it to see that our energy is a finite resource.

I first heard of spoon theory several years ago from a client with ADHD. This concept, created by those with chronic illnesses, describes fluctuating daily energy levels (Raposo 2024). Much like my mystery spoons, every day we wake up with a different number of mental spoons. They represent energy, with each corresponding to how many spoons a single or group of tasks might use up.

Many of my clients are neurodivergent or have chronic health issues. Maybe it's just me attracting "my people" since I also manage autoimmune disease with complex PTSD. Throw in the rollercoaster ride that is perimenopause, and some days I don't have the energy to do much of anything. On many days I barely have enough spoons to get things done, and being able to throw on my favorite everyday Youniform in two minutes means I can feel like a functional human versus a messy blob.

Spoon theory is a simple way of explaining a concept called ego depletion, which is a fancy way of saying willpower. We often think of willpower as something we have control over, making us either weak-minded or strong-minded. But in reality, willpower is a finite resource, and we can easily use it up completing specific tasks.

For me, that looks like *not* doing something I absolutely should be doing. I really don't like to exercise, and I hate to sweat even more. When my babies were little, we attended a fun program called Stroller Strides. I've always joked that regular exercise is not a form of weight loss for me (not arguing the other benefits here), because the energy I spend working out seems to make me hungrier and less able to resist treats. So, after driving thirty minutes one way, working out in the heat and wrangling toddlers, the allure of a Chick-fil-A peach milkshake in the summer was too much to resist. I had already depleted all my willpower, by momming and sweating. Thank goodness I unknowingly had an exercise Youniform in those days too!

What things do you need to say "no" to in the second half of the day? The actual cost of decision fatigue isn't the minutes we spend choosing an outfit; it's the time it steals from us having a purpose-driven day. Overeating, bingeing on sweets, alcohol, getting takeout again, scrolling on your phone, staying up too late...and the list goes on. Temptation is the oldest story around—from the tree of knowledge of good and evil until this very moment—it surrounds us every day. Sometimes we need every single bit of our willpower to avoid that negative thing that is making life worse. Studies show that those with "more" self-control have higher levels of achievement and success

(Gillebaart 2018). Every one of us has a daily to-do list that is filled with big goal tasks and boring required activities.

We can't avoid our daily task list, and even if we can reduce it, putting on clothes is a bit of a necessary evil. But we can reduce the amount of spoons we use for that task. Planning your outfits with the Youniform Framework can help you make less choices each day, which frees up your energy for other things. Be honest with yourself now about how much energy you have on average each day. Do you wake up with your 20-year-old gusto, or is each day a bit of a surprise for how you can go about your daily tasks? Are you skipping things you would like to prioritize because you simply don't have the energy?

We can streamline and systemize much of our day if we do a bit of work upfront to make it easy. Imagine that tomorrow is a significant day for your family: You're about to finalize an investment decision that will set up a future for your children. You spring up with excitement as your alarm rings, knowing that today guides your legacy. You open your closet and, instead of feeling stressed, you feel happy and relaxed because your clothes match who you are now. The rods are filled with groups of clothing for date nights with your hubby of twenty years, cute soccer Saturday options, and a small collection of high-quality important meeting clothes. You know precisely what looks good on your body, even though it's ten pounds heavier than you'd like. You decide on the navy shift dress and emerald green blazer, and pick a pair of navy loafers and jewelry to match. The woman staring back from the mirror is confident and poised, ready to have a day that resonates for generations.

Try this simple experiment: Before you go to bed tonight, decide and lay out your outfit for tomorrow. Stick with it, no matter what mood you wake up in. Notice how it sets up your day with ease and simplicity versus feeling frazzled and frumpy.

How to Dress Like the Woman You're Becoming

Every day that you wake up is a chance to do something amazing. I believe that each of us was put on this earth for a reason. As a person of faith, I have my barometer for what that is and what I am here to do. But each day we follow a drive within us to create something lasting and meaningful. All of us want to know that we left our mark on the world, even if it is only through the people whose lives we changed.

I always find my clients to be such interesting people. Each of them has a different life, but all of them are rich with nuance and texture. It is a gift to get to know each of them and see their triumphs and failures, strengths, and weaknesses. No matter how simple they may feel their life is, every one of them is wonderfully unique in her own way.

Every time you get dressed, you are communicating something. So let's make sure it's what you intend to say.

Like my client Janice, who came to me nearing the end of her military career. She shared her plans to move to Bali to start her own business, but she had no idea what to wear. So I created three powerful Youniforms for her: a work from home outfit with flowy beach colors, an outfit for lounging at the beach and jumping in for a swim, and beautiful activewear for her fitness lifestyle.

Janice's story reminds me that sometimes style changes mark life changes. The clothes aren't the point; the permission is. Once she saw herself as someone free to create a new life, everything else aligned.

Your life is far more meaningful than what you are wearing. Life is bigger than what you are wearing each day. But...you have to get dressed. It's an unavoidable rule of society that we can't go out in public naked. My assistant likes to recall the thing I said that one time that gave her a big revelation:

Every time you get dressed, you are communicating something. So let's make sure it's what you intend to say.

I didn't intend to create a mantra, but it became the catalyst to thinking about style as a powerful way of speaking our inner sense of self.

What you wear isn't about fashion. It's about making life easier so you can focus on what truly matters. It's also sobering because we can get it wrong, and then what divine moments might we be missing? I've heard from women who finally packed a simple Youniform for a marriage retreat and discovered they could show up fully present for the first time in years. Others have shared that feeling comfortable in their clothes freed them to listen when a friend called in a crisis, instead of being distracted by jeans that dug into their stomach.

We miss opportunities too, when low confidence keeps us playing small. One woman landed her dream job after she started wearing a charcoal blazer in her perfect neutral, the same outfit she had once dismissed as too plain. And when we stop worrying about what others think, we show up differently. Another woman said yes to a mom's night out for the first time in years because she finally felt confident instead of frumpy.

These stories may sound small, but they are deeply human. If you've ever stood in front of your mirror on the verge of tears because the person staring back at you feels like a stranger, you know how powerful these shifts can be. We can't hide our self-image and confidence level, good or bad. They always show up in our body language and how we move through the world.

When we have a vision for our life and a purpose, the external bits fall into place. We are no longer reaching and striving to appear to be someone we are not, because our compass is fully aligned on making forward progress to fulfill those goals. We don't care if our clothes are trendy or what designer labels are on them, because our vision for life is so big that those things don't matter.

Take a moment to stop and reflect on the purpose you have for your life. The best way to uncover the truth is to think about the end. How do you want to be remembered? What things do you want people to say about you at your funeral? What kind of person do you hope surfaces as a constant throughout your life? What legacy do you want to leave behind?

When you reflect on what will be left when you are gone, it puts into perspective what you are doing now. Are you living the life of the person you want to be remembered as? What shifts do you need to make to become that person? What milestones do you need to reach in your life to make a beautiful end your reality? I am not a self-help guru or life coach, but these questions always help me reframe who I am, and what I am doing.

When you extrapolate your purpose into your personal style, logic demands that you ask if your clothing is helping you meet that vision. You see that your purpose and vision and destiny are unique. And it frees you to see your outward style as an expression of that one-of-a-kind and fascinating human that you are becoming.

Before you go any further, stop and pull out a piece of paper. (Handwriting makes it stick in the brain). Allow your mind to drift through the questions above and get back in touch with the core of who you are and the woman you want to become. Paint a picture in your mind of what she is doing on a regular day and let your brain fill in the gaps of what she is wearing. Let this become the beginning of your self-discovery of style: meeting the future you and imagining how she embodies her inner self through style.

In the following chapter, we'll uncover the seedy underbelly of the fashion industry, and you'll see how you've been set up to fail. You've been told what to wear your whole life. Next, I'll show you who's been profiting from your confusion and how to take back control of your style.

Chapter One Highlights

- Most women wear only a small fraction of their wardrobes, yet getting dressed consumes outsized time and mental energy.
- The frustration of "nothing to wear" is not a clothing problem, but a decision problem.
- Decision fatigue begins early in the day, long before meaningful work or relationships receive attention.
- Minor, repetitive choices drain finite brainpower and reduce our ability to prioritize what truly matters.
- Automating everyday decisions, especially around clothing, preserves energy for higher-impact choices.
- Simplifying what you wear is not about caring less, but about removing friction so you can live with intention.
- Every time you get dressed, you are communicating something, whether you realize it or not.

Two

The Perfect Closet

"Only those who will risk going too far can possibly find out how far one can go." — T.S. Eliot

Facebook® was working hard the day it served me the done-for-you capsule wardrobe ad. A great graphic showed a spreadsheet-style page with images of different clothing put together into outfits that required no thinking. I was sold. My capsule wardrobe fantasy was about to become reality.

I bought the paid program, made my own spreadsheet of every single clothing item (around sixty-five) and started collecting every piece. I followed the suggestions religiously, putting together each outfit as suggested, even when my internal voice was screaming at me.

I figured that after four kids (and pregnant with a fifth), the person who created this guide surely knew more than me, since she was running a business on the idea. At that time, of course she did. As I purchased item after item because it was recommended, I stopped listening to the part of myself who knew a definite no. I was in the experimentation phase, and I went all out.

I spent a large amount of money gathering every recommended item, and sometimes the first version didn't work, so I kept trying. I kept telling myself that it must be *me* and I needed to make every single item work because this lady said it was stylish. As time went on, I became unsettled because I kept defaulting to the same outfit types (hello early Youniforms). Everyone said I needed a variety of outfits, and wearing the same thing on repeat felt like a failure. But the experience ended up giving me more knowledge in the long run.

I thought my experience was unique to me, and that I must be some outlier, but over the years, I've talked to dozens of other women in my online communities that had the exact same experience. They bought clothes that were standardized by someone else, curated on paper to look great, and realized that their style was different. Over half of them had at least $200 worth of unworn clothes in their closets. Just like me, they felt silly and embarrassed every time they looked at the wasted money hanging in their closets, many with tags still dangling, destined never to be worn.

See, I was seeking the "perfect" capsule wardrobe, and I was determined to have it. For years this meant collecting other people's ideas of perfection. From fast fashion to influencer culture to done-for-you solutions, we are inundated with other people's ideas of what makes an ideal capsule wardrobe.

In this chapter, I want to share how the fashion cycle has been hijacked and accelerated, and why you, as the consumer, must learn to lean into your own style instead of listening to the marketing propaganda. By the end, you'll see why most of us are helpless against the onslaught of the fashion industry, and you'll have a new perspective on the clothes in your closet.

When Clothing Stopped Being Valuable

I took home economics in ninth grade, and the first thing I remember sewing on a machine was a scrunchie for my hair. Then came pajama pants out of woven cotton for my final grade. The craft and creativity of sewing stuck with me, and after my second child was born, I had a small business sewing boutique girls' dresses. The process of creating a garment from fabric gives the mind time to think due to the monotony of the process: cut the pattern pieces, pin them together, create seams, open and iron the seams, attach the next piece until the garment is complete, and then add the finishing touches like buttons or trim. Each dress I created took multiple hours from start to finish, and I charged over $50 for toddler items.

For one single dress, I invested hours of my labor plus the cost of materials. Even cheap fabric is $2-3 per yard, and the cost of small materials like thread, facings, buttons, and the like adds up quickly. If you assume just $10 for materials for one child's garment, then add on four hours of labor at minimum wage, the cost to produce is already at $38. This doesn't include things like freight, quality control, or lost inventory that occurs for a large company.

This is just a small snapshot into the process of creating clothing. But when you take a look at the average closet, you see dozens (if not hundreds) of pieces on the rack. Walk into a modern clothing store, and you are overwhelmed with choices, and that's not even accounting for online shopping like Shein and Amazon. The term for this modern style of clothing is called fast fashion,

(1) because it is actually produced quickly and (2) because it isn't made to last.

For most of history, clothing was a high-item expense in a family's budget. The entire process was done by hand, often by women or children hand spinning or weaving fabric. The biblical Proverbs 31 woman illustrates this as a king's wife:

- "She looks for wool and linen..." (Proverbs 31:13 [New American Standard Bible] which shows the gathering of materials.

- "She stretches out her hands to the distaff, and her hands grasp the spindle" (Proverbs 31:19 [NASB]) using spinning and weaving tools.

- She uses expensive dyes: "...clothed with scarlet" (Proverbs 31:20 [NASB]) and "clothing is fine linen and purple" (Proverbs 31:21 [NASB]).

Each person typically only had a few garments, and because of the high cost, these were mended and passed down to last as long as possible. As fashion emerged after the Renaissance because of industrialization and trade, it was still only the wealthiest who could afford these new and novel styles, while the middle and lower classes maintained a few items. Even as inventions developed that sped up the time needed to harvest, spin yarn, and weave fabrics, tailors still did the construction of garments by hand.

For example, linen is one of the oldest fabrics to be found in historical records. We can examine the development of a single linen garment found in ancient civilizations to see the origins of the clothes we wear. Before it can become linen fabric, it begins as a seed that grows into the flax plant. Once grown, it's best harvested by hand to maintain the most fiber, which is found inside the stalk (stem) of the plant. At this point, a weeks-long process begins to separate out the usable portion of the flax that will become linen (Addad 2022). These are individual fibers, like an individual strand of hair, which must then be spun into yarn. The yarn is then woven into the final finished fabric, notwithstanding any dyeing that occurs. Finally, the fabric is cut and sewn into a garment, a tunic in historical times, which was then gathered and held to the body by various types of fasteners or ties.

This is a lot of technical background, but for us today this history matters. We have strayed so far from the true cost of clothing that most of us no longer understand what actually goes into making clothes. $5 shirts can easily convince us that the process is cheap or inexpensive.

The Youniform Framework shows you how to be intentional, ensuring every purchase lasts for years.

But it was the invention of the sewing machine in 1846 that changed the trajectory of fashion forever (Stefanie 2019). Initially invented a decade before to speed up production of military uniforms, the sewing machine took a process that was done by hand slowly and methodically and turned it into a seam that can be completed in a few seconds. Near the end of the 19th century, *ready-to-wear* clothing was available in catalogs and department stores in the United States, forever changing how people buy clothing.

By the mid-20th century, many clothing stores opened to meet this growing trend, and the wealth boom after World War II contributed to the desire for easier access to clothing.

The self-expression of style through fashion—once only available to the ultra-wealthy and nobility—became a part of everyday life. With it, the demand for more clothing, faster, encouraged companies to shift their manufacturing to Asia, where the cycle grew teeth because of low wages and fewer restrictions on working conditions and safety. The term "fast fashion" first appeared in a New York Times article in 1989 when they did a piece on how Zara takes clothes from factory floor to store in two weeks (Nizzoli 2024).

Nowadays, the global fashion industry is worth around $1.84 trillion and employs almost 12% of the global workforce (Cardona 2025). Mass manufacturing plants mean that clothing can be created in minutes versus the hours of one person doing it by hand. But fast fashion is a fairly new concept, even within the full view of history, that has only arisen within the last fifty years to be the mammoth industry it is today.

This massive shift in clothing production has fundamentally changed how we think about fashion. These days we think nothing of buying brand new inexpensive clothing on a whim, but for 99% of history, clothing was considered a precious commodity to own. Even after clothing moved to industry, there were still just two seasons of production for hundreds of years.

Even though your grandmother bought mass-produced clothing, she only did it twice a year. Those purchases were considered thoughtfully, and quality items were purchased. They had less clothing in their closets, meaning less decision fatigue. When their garments showed signs of wear, they often mended before replacing them.

But now, each week is a new season of trends, and each piece is only intended to last for a couple of wash and wears. We have been conditioned to think we should shop for clothes every month, and some people even shop every day. Instead of figuring out how to love and get more use out of what we already have, we forget about it with the next shopping dopamine hit.

Fast fashion means that we've lost the ability to appreciate clothing for its function but also for the craftsmanship that used to go into its creation. It has also caused us to lose our own sense of self-expression, as we often buy because of influence or marketing, rather than intentional personal choice.

But the Youniform Framework shifts the power back into your hands and shows you how to be intentional, ensuring every purchase lasts for years. Think about the last clothing item you purchased and answer these questions:

- When did you buy it?
- What was the price?
- How many times have you worn it?
- What is the cost-per-wear (price divided by number of times worn)?
- How long will you likely keep it?
- On a scale of 1 to 5, with 5 being completely in love, how do you feel about it?

When my clients do this exercise, they are always a bit shocked...for a few items, cost per wear is nearly nothing and they rate it four or five. But for most of their closets, the cost per wear is over $20 and they don't even know why they bought it. This is one of the many strengths of a Youniform: building a closet with at least 90% items you'd rate a five.

The history of fashion is an intriguing journey, and industrialization has forever changed the way we shop and dress. But these moves in the mid-20th century give way to a more sinister issue in your closet.

The Human Cost of Modern Fashion

In 2001, I walked into Express for the first time and left with a $60 leopard print off the shoulder top in chiffon. Other than formal wear, it was the most expensive single item of clothing I had ever purchased for myself. I wore that shirt nearly every night out with my friends and kept it for years before finally donating it in my late 20s. At the time, it represented financial independence and made me feel grown up every time I wore it (even though in reality I was a train wreck of a young adult).

I wore that top constantly. It followed me through nights out, different seasons of life, and eventually even styled with a jacket for work. I kept it for years simply because I loved it enough to keep reaching for it. I finally donated it with a pang of regret because the elastic had stretched out from being worn so often that it no longer fit correctly. Shopping used to be like this...a hunt for a gorgeous item, excitement at the score, joy when wearing it on repeat, and holding on to it for nearly a decade.

But for many people, the shopping experience has changed.

And the pandemic of 2020 rewrote the rules for everyone.

I haven't done in-person shopping since at least the 2020 pandemic, and likely for several years before. The rise of online shopping and major companies like Amazon has made fast fashion easily accessible. Influencer trends like video shopping hauls with dozens of unboxings in one single haul, try-on sessions of twenty or thirty different tops, and 'shop my link' show us a world where the cool people are buying new clothes constantly, all at low, low prices. Whether it's a $15 trending top at Walmart or Target or $20 jeans on Amazon, clothing prices have never been more accessible.

But what if I told you that the inexpensive shirt you're wearing right now is possibly a death sentence?

By the time an item of clothing is placed in a store for sale, it has become a world traveler. The raw materials are grown or created in one part of the world, shipped to another to be made into fabric, sent to yet another to be sewn, and again elsewhere to be dyed and trimmed, then crossed oceans to warehouses all over the planet, and finally to individual retail locations. Each step of the journey costs money, and when considering a cheap item, fractions of a dollar go into each part of the journey on a piece of clothing that is typically marked up at 50%. The only way to make this feasible is to keep the pieces of clothing production housed in places where the cost is less regulated.

In fact, at the time of this writing we are seeing volatile discussions of tariffs, and I have personally witnessed a small Christian clothing brand say that if they brought manufacturing to our home country that the prices of one item would triple to over $300. This statement should raise the question of how we can access millions of pieces of clothing daily that are so incredibly cheap. The answer is that clothing manufacturing is primarily done in parts of the world where there are minimal or no regulations in environmental and manufacturing safety. Most of the clothing in industrialized nations comes from garment-producing nations in Asia (India, China, Vietnam, Bangladesh are the top producers). (Kennemer 2025) But in these countries, no one bats an eye at pollution or worker safety, so the factories continue working. But what is it really like to be a garment worker?

Of the over seventy-five million garment workers around the world (most of whom are women), only 2% earn a living wage. (Helm 2024) A living wage is the minimum cost necessary to cover basic necessities like housing, food, clothing, and healthcare with a buffer for unexpected expenses. Around the world, this minimum number varies between developed countries (~$3000/mo) and poorer nations ($570/mo in Vietnam). But the average wage for garment workers is often less than half needed to meet these needs. When these workers try to protest or unionize, they are punished and their efforts ignored.

The bustling capital of Bangladesh, megacity Dhaka, is one of the most densely populated cities in the world with over ten million people. People come from the villages to the city to secure employment at low wages and long hours. Textiles are one of the top ten industries, with women flocking to this form of employment.

Like in most major cities, buildings shoot up into the sky, reflecting the limited land space and demand to build upward. An eight-story building blends seamlessly into the industrial landscape. On the first floor, it houses shops and banks, and on the remaining levels, various garment factories. On April 23rd, 2013, dangerous cracks were noticed throughout the building, and it was declared unsafe, and those inside told to leave.

The bottom levels closed, but the following morning, the garment workers received calls from their supervisors to return to work. Fearing the loss of their jobs and livelihood, over 3,500 headed back into the dangerous building.

When the rumbling began, many immediately ran for the exits, some jumping out the window onto other structures. As the concrete broke and collapsed in a cloud of dust, thousands were trapped under debris. The stories of 2,500 survivors tell of amputated limbs, crushed spines, the loss of fertility, traumatic brain injury with lifelong disability, and so much more.

But for 1,134 souls, the *story just ends.*

After twenty days of recovery efforts, the search was called off. Rescue workers later shared stories of the permeating smell of decay of bodies trapped in the rubble.

Rana Plaza is one of the deadliest industrial disasters *of all time.* But if you think it's just cheap brands that were involved, you'd be wrong.

Most of the clothes being made inside were for big brands in developed countries: Benetton (Italy), Cato Fashions (USA), JC Penney (USA), Mango (Spain), Primark (UK), The Children's Place (USA), and Walmart (USA), plus twenty-four other brands you'd probably recognize (Clean Clothes Campaign 2015). Despite revenues in the millions and billions, most of the families have received little to no compensation for their disability and loss. The financial hunger of the mighty fashion industry has never been more pronounced than in this incident.

And while tragedies like this grab the spotlight and help make small changes in clothing production, a similar story of danger and disability is happening in thousands of factories around the world. From factory fires, to limb injuries, to declining health from chemical runoff, the fashion industry profits off of $20 items only because it can produce them for less than half of that in regulated countries.

When I first read the list of companies linked to Rana Plaza, the building that collapsed in Bangladesh, I saw a couple I had shopped. The Children's Place jumped out at me as a regular go-to for affordable kids' clothes. I was appalled to realize I had been clothing my kids in leggings that might have cost someone their life.

Curious to see if they have changed any practices since 2013, I checked the app Good on You, which is an app that ranks companies on their ethical and safety practices. In 2021 The Children's Place received a grading of "poor" by the Fashion Transparency Index and they still don't engage in certified labor standards. I checked the labels on the clothes I have here at home and found they were manufactured in Ethiopia.

The first step is awareness. I'm not going to ask you never again to buy $5 kids shorts, because sometimes that's the best option for your sensory-sensitive child. But perhaps just knowing where your clothes come from can help. As we end this section, I'd love for you to consider your favorite brand and do the following:

- Go to their website and check their About Us or Sustainability page.
- Check a few labels of items you own and see where they were made.
- Check Good on You or do a Google search "brand name + factory workers" and see what comes up.
- Take note of the average worker's wage in the countries you found, and any surprising info you learned in the process.

It would take a massive reframing of fashion worldwide to change how we use clothing, specifically fast fashion.

"Know better, do better"...now that I know this information, I can't stick my head in the sand, and hopefully neither can you. But we can be mindful and try to make better choices when possible about how we consume clothes and how we use our money.

Why Expensive Doesn't Mean Quality

Back before easy sites like Poshmark and Mercari, you had to do your thrifting on sites like eBay (which is an amazing stealth source for secondhand clothes). Months before my very first cruise, my college budget had me scouring it for the perfect clothes to take with me. When I found a navy French terry swim cover-up with a little horse logo on the left chest, still with tags, I squealed with delight. In my mind, Ralph Lauren Polo was synonymous with an upper-class style that I typically couldn't afford.

Emboldened by my find, this marked the start of building my closet with previously inaccessible brands with some extra time and research effort. But what is our obsession with labels and luxury brands, and where did it all begin? And...are they even that much better than a similar shirt with a no-name label?

Caste systems permeate history; from the French Revolution to the British aristocracy, humans have always wanted to be part of the wealthy classes. Class systems are still alive and well today, even in countries you might not expect, like the United States, and exist across the world in various ways.

But fashion is one area where even those of little means can buy something from an expensive brand, and people can use clothes as a status symbol to aspire to a higher social class. The idea of dressing well for the upper class began in 1858 with the origination of *haute couture.*

Haute couture, which means "high fashion" in French, finds its beginning with Charles Frederick Worth (of the fashion house, the House of Worth) who changed the landscape of style in Paris by incorporating live models, seasonal collections, and sewing labels into garments (Edwards 2024). The ultra-wealthy and nobility would visit his home, where they would be measured and custom garments created just for them. The process birthed other legacy high fashion brands like Dior and Chanel.

As the demand for these prestigious designers increased, many brands launched "ready-to-wear" collections to give more people access to their creations. If you've seen *The Devil Wears Prada*, then you know what's coming. The one-of-a-kind creations that walk the runway create a trickle-down trend effect until knockoffs and copies appear in discount retailers like Walmart, Target, Amazon, or Shein. It's called the fashion pyramid and shows how different brands fit into the landscape of the fashion industry.

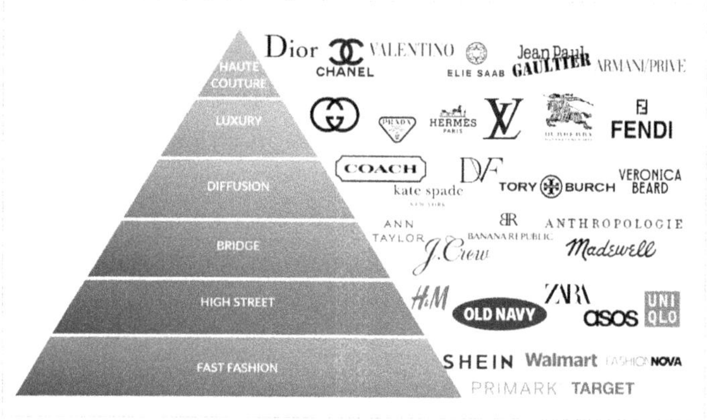

Figure 2.1 Fashion pyramid showing different brand placement from fast fashion to haute couture (for full color images visit youniformbook.com).

It's the labels that we all recognize now, like my delight about the Polo horse on the swim coverup. I'm sure you can easily picture iconic symbols like those of Louis Vuitton or Prada. And wearing these is all about aspiration: about achieving a status recognized by others, that is typically afforded to the wealthy, which is funny since those with generational wealth rarely wear anything with a visible label. Natural scarcity perpetuates this (like a Birkin bag), but higher price points compound the exclusivity. You would expect these designer items to be of the highest quality, based on reputation and price, but that is frequently not the case.

If you were to peek at a Versace label, you would expect to see "made in Italy" and you very well might. But brands are allowed to offshore most of their production, bring the product home for small finishes, and slap a home source of origin. It's misleading, and as previously discussed, we would expect the low-wage countries to produce mostly discount goods, but a 2014 report found that the same factory in Moldova was producing discount brand garments alongside those from Versace, Dolce & Gabbana, and Armani (Hoskins 2014). Going further, you can examine the fabric content and trace the source materials to see that it's all coming from the same place. Ultimately, the only difference between a white button-down shirt from Walmart and one from Ralph Lauren is the label sewn inside (and the price).

There's a saying I love, "wealth whispers," and you can see this often in the multi-millionaires and their daily choices. From simple cars to understated tees, they often choose quality items without labels. Indeed in some parts of the world, like Europe, adorning oneself in labels to show off is considered bad taste. Outside of red carpet events or actual royalty, those obsessed with certain brands are often doing so to garner prestige and influence from those around them. When you realize that an actual knockoff was produced right next to the real deal, the sheen of ascending through fashion fades a bit. And for women looking to live a life of legacy and impact, the moments in our clothes matter far more than the labels *on* our clothes.

I'm no longer obsessed with Polo, and have found that my attempts at shopping for these "bridge brands"—brands that "bridge" the wealth gap—often leave me disgusted when I look into the quality and composition.

I would like to challenge your perception of brands. Consider a brand that you equate with luxury and aspire to attain. Why does this brand have this effect on you? Would you still enjoy the exact same item if it had a different label? How would it feel if you had a wardrobe filled with high-quality items from brands that are unrecognizable other than their reputation?

How to Buy Clothes that Last

If brand names don't define the quality of a garment, what does? It's also not dependent on price, although no-name brands often confer better products per price point than vanity brands. Quality is defined as the degree of excellence of something, and when it comes to clothing, can be identified by construction and material. Construction can be harder to judge, especially since high-end clothing is often made in the same factories as discount clothing. Imagine two blazers, one that is of true high quality and one that is of cheap quality.

- Inferior quality: single layer, polyester blend. Shoulder seams bulge and lift, sleeves are slightly different lengths, seams have exposed raw edges created with an overlock machine, button threads are loose.
- High quality: wool blend, lined. Shoulder seams align on the body, all the seams are hidden, the bodice has darts to improve fit, and buttonholes are even and precise.

In the realm of garment construction, more detail often means more precision, but it depends on the quality standards of the factory. Since this aspect is slightly harder to control as a consumer, the biggest quality marker is often fabric type.

There are two classes of fabrics: natural and synthetic, and the rest of this section is dedicated to explaining the difference between the two. In its simplest definition, natural fibers are those that are plant or animal based, and synthetic fibers are those created by chemical processes. Natural fibers have been the dominant material in clothing for most of the history of humanity. As explored earlier in this chapter, this process is labor-intensive, but yields fabric that is durable and breathable. Below you'll find the most common types of natural fibers, along with their characteristics and basic info.

FIBER	SOURCE	COMMON NAMES	TYPE	KEY TRAITS
COTTON	COTTON PLANT PODS	EGYPTIAN/ SUPIMA	WOVEN & KNIT	BREATHABLE AND MOISTURE WICKING
LINEN	FLAX PLANT STEM	BELGIAN LINEN	WOVEN	EXCEPTIONAL BREATHABILITY & HIGH FREQUENCY
HEMP	CANNABIS PLANT STEM	--	WOVEN	BREATHABLE & MOISTURE WICKING
WOOL	SHEEP/GOAT FLEECE	MERINO/CASHMERE/ LAMBSWOOL	WOVEN & KNIT	HEAT RETAINING AND MOISTURE WICKING
SILK	SILKWORM THREAD	MULBERRY/ SHANTUNG/ DUPIONI	WOVEN (BIAS CUT)	BREATHABLE AND MOISTURE WICKING
ANGORA/MO HAIR/ALPACA	VARIES	--	WOVEN & KNIT	HEAT RETAINING AND MOISTURE WICKING

Table 2.2 Common types of natural fibers showing source, names, use, and features.

Natural fibers are increasingly hard to find, but most retailers publish fabric content for their garments, and cotton, silk, and wool can be found in many mass-market stores. Some companies are dedicated to producing garments in one category of natural fiber, and these small businesses usually have loyal followings and make quality clothing. All the natural fibers mesh well with the human body, most providing moisture wicking (anti sweat) properties, superior breathability which prevents yeast and bacteria buildup on the skin, and many are more durable and require less laundering. It's likely because these materials come from nature, where a plant must be hardy to survive full growth and animal fur must be able to withstand dirt and the elements. When we sustainably turn these into clothing, we get the benefits of God's creation in nature.

Synthetic fibers—like polyester, Lycra, nylon, spandex, viscose, rayon, acrylic, and acetate—are made by refining petrochemicals like oil and gas into wearable fibers. This process originated in the late 19th century with the first faux silk. DuPont Chemical revolutionized the synthetic fiber industry in 1935 with the creation of nylon. Used in everything from pantyhose to wartime parachutes, the advent of industrialized fabric creation changed the landscape of fashion. Polyester was introduced in the 1950s and is now found in over 50% of clothing produced worldwide (Galloway 2024).

When we return to our roots, own less clothing and value it more, we open the door to joy in more meaningful areas of life.

While the accessibility of synthetic fabric is unchallenged, it is inferior to natural fibers in most ways. It suffers from the typical critiques of the petroleum industry, from environmental concerns to health issues of workers. Recent research also suggests a growing concentration of microplastics in human brains, which stems from the massive use of plastics in daily life (Nihart et al. 2025). We may not realize that synthetic garments shed large amounts of microplastics with every wash cycle, and since they lack the wicking and reusability of natural fibers, this typically happens with every wear.

Adopting natural fibers into your wardrobe is one of the best ways to increase the quality without spending thousands on designer goods. The benefit of this transition is that your clothes last longer because you wash them less and they are more durable. Your body will also thank you as it learns again to breathe without stifling plastic disguised as fabric. Finally, switching to natural fiber clothing leads to owning less, because you begin to appreciate the inherent luxury of clothing designed by nature to suit your life. I encourage all clients to aim for at least 50% natural fiber composition on all garments, to ensure they are getting the best possible items with enhanced longevity.

You may be surprised to see what your clothes are made of. I invite you to explore your clothes and check the labels. See what fibers are in your closet, and research how each is made. We take for granted the clothes we wear, a modern luxury of abundance, but clothing was once prized as a luxury item for most people.

When we return to our roots, own less clothing and value it more, we open the door to joy in more meaningful areas of life.

Clothes Don't Die Quietly

Even natural fibers don't last forever, so what happens to clothing when we are done with it?

Your favorite shirt has outlived its usefulness to you, and assuming it isn't damaged or stained, you put it in the donate box, dropping it off at Goodwill or your local charity. Many of us believe that the clothing gets washed and put on the floor for local resale, but only 10-15% ends up being used in this way (Tonti 2025). What happens to the other 90% may be shocking.

First, the clothes are sorted to determine what should stay and what should go. Your local secondhand store or charity sends the unused clothing to sorting centers, where mass quantities of discarded clothes are sorted. The good quality stuff that didn't have a home locally may get sent to vintage stores around the country. But the majority is bundled and packaged to be sent out into the global secondhand market. Most of these clothes end up in Africa, Asia, or Eastern European countries, often clogging beaches or eradicating a local artisan clothing market. In some places the secondhand fashion is welcomed as these nations don't have access to the same modern fashions as the first world. But many times, our discards are sent away to be someone else's trash problem. Graphic images show clothing littering the beaches of Ghana, polluting coral reef systems and piling up in deserts in Chile (James 2022).

Back at the sorting warehouse, the stuff that didn't make the cut still has two outcomes: textile recycling or trash. Textile recycling or downcycling is when a fabric item is broken down from its original design and turned into a lesser item like a rag or stuffing. Less than 1% of clothing textiles are reused in new clothing items (Brown 2023). But this is actually something we could do at home: repurposing old clothing into cleaning cloths or finding another solution.

But what of the rest of the unwearable and unwanted clothing that is destined for disposal? The final resting place of clothing is either the landfill or an incinerator, but each has its own drawbacks. Remember that most of the clothing we wear is synthetic, and even many natural fiber items are mixed with small amounts of nylon or spandex to make them more wearable.

In each disposal instance, the clothing we wear becomes an environmental nightmare.

Landfills are so filled with discarded clothes they form mountains. Like a large fabric compost pile, but a melting pot of natural and synthetic fibers. The natural fibers will eventually break down, releasing methane gas as they return to the earth. But the synthetic fibers will last hundreds of years, finally breaking down into microplastics, which leach into the soil and groundwater.

Incineration is a faster disposal technique, but is far less used and mostly limited to parts of Europe. It's still a source of greenhouse emissions of carbon dioxide and methane, along with toxic chemicals from synthetic clothing. Nearby villagers are often ill from the smoke released from these clothing incinerators.

It is estimated that the amount of discarded clothing per person per year is 85lb, or the equivalent of an average 10-year-old (Igini 2023). Each of us is responsible for this process in a cycle of buy fast and donate faster. Most clothing now is not made to last for multiple generations, but is worn a few times and discarded for the next shiny thing.

The question becomes: how can we reduce our disposal and consumption and reconsider clothing to be an investment rather than a hobby or habit?

Obviously, you can buy less and make better choices, which is the focus of this book. You can also thrift for vintage or like-new items. Learn how to make small hidden repairs on your quality clothing items. Research sustainable clothing recycling near you and stop dropping off your items at Goodwill. Find a way to reuse, recycle, and buy less.

Distance doesn't negate the impact your choices are having. Feeding money back into unethical fashion is actively harming people you've never met on the other side of the world. And you can't change the world...but as one person you can influence one more and start a chain reaction. Our clothing literally affects the entire world, and we get to be a positive change when we reframe our approach away from collecting clothes for the sake of having more variety.

But the fashion industry is only the beast outside the door; we also have to face the voice inside our head telling us we're not good enough, and in the next chapter, we're going to tackle that beast together.

Chapter Two Highlights

- The "perfect closet" is usually someone else's idea of style, not something designed around your real body or life.
- Fast fashion changed clothing from a valued resource into something disposable, cheap, and easily replaced.
- Low clothing prices are only possible because the real costs are paid by workers, communities, and the environment.
- Brand names and high prices do not guarantee quality, since luxury and discount clothing are often made the same way.
- Fabric and construction matter more than labels, with natural fibers lasting longer and working better with the body.
- The Youniform Framework refocuses the goal from having more clothes to owning fewer pieces you actually love and wear.

Three

Just One Dress

"Simplicity is the keynote of all true elegance." - Coco Chanel

The lowest moment in my style journey is the most revealing. I've probably told the following story a hundred times, but it remains the reason I'm sharing any of this with you now.

It was 2020, the year of the pandemic, and we were deep in lockdown mode in the summer. My fifth baby came late with his embodied drama, causing me endless amounts of stress. He was later than all the others (well past forty weeks), kept me in active labor for five days, and came out covered head to toe in meconium. At twenty-four hours old, his blood sugar bottomed out, and we had to supplement with formula. It took two solid weeks before he ever developed the milk-drunk look.

I was a mess in every way: physically from having a newborn at thirty-nine, emotionally with all the postpartum hormones, and mentally with lockdowns and a hard baby. To add insult to injury,

I had an autoimmune flare almost immediately after he was born, and my skin was numb in some places or too sensitive in others.

My outfit experiments ended abruptly. I'm an advocate of loungewear in the fourth trimester postpartum, but when I started trying to wear real clothes, things fell apart quickly. It was all horribly uncomfortable. I hated the way sleeves felt on my arms, and anything with a hard waist made me feel like crawling out of my skin. I was down to pajamas or a dress.

Needing to get dressed occasionally for my mental health, I kept choosing dresses. I had a decent collection of nursing dresses, and I added more because it was easy and simple. Occasionally, I would try a different outfit variation, and disgusted, I would take it off faster than I put it on.

One day I had a random thought, and as a verbal processor, I turned to my husband to see if I was a genius or an idiot.

"Hey, do you think I could just wear the same dress every day in different colors, and maybe this same cardigan...and that could be my entire wardrobe?"

His look confirmed that I was thinking smart, but also that I had said something very obvious to him.

"Yeah, sure," he said. "I literally asked you to buy me seven of the exact same blue shirt."

Inside my head, it was like the ball dropping at Times Square, angels singing *Hallelujah*, and a blast of recognition that somewhere inside me, I had *always* known this very simple concept.

Just one dress outfit was absolutely enough...I didn't need fifty different outfit variations. Which brings up the question of why we're so obsessed with variety and having a different outfit for every occasion. Is this something that's just been sold to us, rather than us naturally wanting it?

I actually felt a little foolish at that moment, not because the idea was new, but because it finally crystallized. I already knew this; I had just been overcomplicating it. Instead of cycling through endless outfit combinations, chasing variety, I really just needed cohesion. Maybe that sounds too simple. You might even feel skeptical reading this. But if getting dressed feels harder than it should, it's worth asking whether the issue is a lack of options, or an *excess* of them.

In this chapter we're going to discuss the spotlight effect, why we're obsessed with new clothes all the time, how trend hopping is killing your style, the power of your favorite things, and how wearing what you love builds confidence.

No One Notices What You're Wearing (Seriously)

There's a voice in my head sometimes when I get dressed that says, "You can't wear that; you wore it the last time you went to dinner with friends." That voice is a big fat liar. Many (I'd argue most) of us are consumed with thoughts about how other people perceive us. This extends from the way we look to the car we drive and the house we live in, to the job we have and how our kids act in public. We expect that every person we meet is silently judging every aspect of who we are.

And there is likely some truth there, but people are far more concerned with themselves and what's in their own head than what's going on with you (Carnegie 1936). Style and clothing fall into a funny place in this area, because it's both a powerful form of communication *and* something that isn't often noticed the way we think it is.

There's a psychological principle here called the Spotlight Effect. This is a cognitive bias that leads us to overestimate the amount of attention others are paying to us. It tricks us into thinking *we* are the center of attention, like a performer under a spotlight. We think our friends are going to remember that we wore the same shirt a month ago to brunch, but sometimes even the people closest to us don't notice when we wear the same things. In our preoccupation with our own main character energy, we think we're the main character to everyone else.

A year after I embraced just one dress style to make my life easier, I decided to try the 100-Day Dress Challenge from the sustainable brand Wool&. I had heard of this concept a few years before from a client and it sounded intriguing, but also... a little ridiculous. Wool& created the challenge as a brand awareness campaign: wear the *exact same dress* from their company for 100 days and take photographic evidence. The intended purpose is to promote slow fashion, natural fibers, and anti-consumerism. The reward at the end is a gift card to buy another dress.

As you learned in Chapter Two, natural fibers like merino wool in these dresses hold up well to repeated wearing without repeated laundering. Thousands of women have completed this challenge (myself included) and have walked away with a new appreciation for the simplicity of wearing less. But one of the big questions that comes up is whether anyone noticed.

A couple of years ago I was preparing a workshop on capsule wardrobes and polled this vast community of challenge women on their experiences of being noticed. I have read hundreds of threads over the years from women who kept their 100-Day Dress Challenge a secret from their husband, or even wore a red dress, or got called out for wearing a lot of black, but I wanted to collect these stories to really see if any of these women were affected by repeating the exact same clothing every day. I got over 200 responses, and here are just a few of the highlights:

- One woman, a city commissioner, wore the same black dress unstyled for 100 days, appearing on TV three times a month...and no one noticed.
- Another who did the 100 days, then three more short challenges as a teacher, and not a single student realized.
- Multiple stories of rich red, bright pink, and deep purple dresses that went unnoticed by husbands.
- A woman who only told her husband, then vacationed with her kids and extended family for three weeks...none of whom noticed.

There are tons of stories just like this from a challenge that many would consider extreme, and they all affirm one thing: No one is really noticing what you wear. We spend an inordinate amount of time obsessing over what to wear, trying to keep it new and fresh for fear someone will call us out for repeating an outfit, but it's just a waste of time. We're wasting our lives worrying about something that is proven to have no bearing in reality. Everyone is simply too preoccupied with their own lives, including obsessing over their own clothes, to care about yours.

I can admittedly say that even as a stylist whose job is to critique and focus on people's clothing, I still don't pay attention. I notice the massive faux pas when out and about and have a general sense of what is happening collectively with style, but when I see my friends, I don't remember what they're wearing. I'm too busy enjoying the moment and the connection.

I want you to try this experiment. Consider your closest friend and remember the last time you got together. See if you can remember what they were wearing. If you can, it's probably because there was something that stood out. Go a step further, reach out and tell them you're doing a personal experiment, and ask them if they can remember what they were wearing. If you're embarrassed, you can always say you realized you loved their shirt/pants/dress and ask where they got it. If you're feeling really brave now, ask them if they remember what *you* were wearing. Nine times out of ten, they will not have any idea.

When you can free yourself from thinking that other people are always noticing what you wear, you can embrace a style that is authentically you. The spotlight effect proves that no one notices and no one really cares. Not only can you be free to wear what brings you joy and simplifies your life, but you become untethered to society's expectations about what you should wear.

How Comparison Culture Hijacked Personal Style

One goal of the 100-Day Dress Challenge and other similar style challenges is to illustrate the concept of slow fashion. Previously, we discussed the problems with fast fashion, and slow fashion is a rising trend of people trying to reduce overconsumption. From the deadstock designer in the northern US to a company that sells a five-item capsule wardrobe, people all over the world are turning away from clothing overconsumption. But how did our love affair with shopping hauls and influencer culture even begin?

If you're anything like me, you probably fondly remember collecting fashion or style magazines when you were younger. *Seventeen* magazine was my jam, followed by *Cosmopolitan* once I was officially an adult and ready for the racy articles. I used to buy fresh magazines and spend hours reading them at home, going through the articles, seeing the new items, and looking at the Polo ads. Before the internet revolution, access to style was limited to trickle-down from the top echelon of fashion society. Much like that cerulean clip from *The Devil Wears Prada*, the industry *told* us what to wear. There was an element of gatekeeping, and only the fashion magazines and twice-yearly industry shows gave access to the masses.

But just like all things, the birth of the internet changed forever how we consume fashion. I started blogging before it was a thing, but while others were sharing their love of *stuff*, I was writing horrible poetry and word vomiting my feelings about being dumped by another boyfriend. But savvy stylish individuals who jumped on the train in the early 2000s built enormous wealth as style bloggers. As YouTube took off, many of those written stylistas transitioned to video format. With such a powerful medium to communicate, fashion hauls grew into a frenzy.

A shopping haul is a documentary-style presentation where the individual (male or female) shows off a large number of items that they have bought, often in a single shopping trip. They unbox them, try them on, talk about the features and what they love or hate, and squeal in excitement if they got a good deal. Over time, brands realized that these everyday grassroots movements were actually selling their clothes.

The *influence* of normal people carried more weight than models who lived an ideal life.

And so, influencer culture was born. Making money to post cute outfits and talk about things you like seems like easy money. Indeed, a recent poll showed that most of Gen Alpha's aspirational career goals were related to content creation or influencing (Burleigh 2025). But while many are making money through influencing, and the brands certainly take advantage of that user-generated content, this shift from controlled fashion information to influencer overwhelm has had a massive impact on what we view as "normal."

Our kids get brand new stuff for birthdays and Christmas, and I manage a list for each kid for extended family to shop as well. Once a month they are allowed to look at their list, delete items, and add new stuff. But one of our children is obsessed with looking at his Amazon wishlist. So much so that even on my password-locked phone, I'll sometimes catch him peeking at the list.

So, my husband and I have conversations on end with this one son, who really loves window shopping, always trying to drive home the lesson to him that constantly focusing on things you don't have causes constant dissatisfaction with the things you do. But even Holly Golightly loved to window shop, standing at Tiffany's with her croissant and coffee. I think the classic story shows many of the downsides of lusting too much.

Influencer culture is perfectly targeted to flip that switch, and when you scroll a feed and see ad after ad, gorgeous woman after another modeling clothing, it's hard not to want to take a bite. The nature of the demanding culture and subtle message to "never be seen twice in that" means the quality of the promoted items is getting lower.

Teenagers on a budget doing a haul have to source from places like SHEIN or Amazon. More fast fashion that's just going to end up in a landfill, all to make the corporations happy.

An upper middle-class mom is often hustling Old Navy or Gap to keep the price point low for her audience. And these don't last much longer.

As you already know; cheap crap doesn't last.

The fabric is fake, the construction is shoddy, the quality is second rate, and the style itself is temporary. Influencer culture should be called *throwaway culture.*

But these (usually) gorgeous women play games with our minds as well. It's more than "look at this great jacket I found for $50." It's also "See my newly remodeled kitchen, or my subtle lip injections, or the diet I follow to stay slim, or my kid's achievements (which are obviously a reflection of my parenting)." Social media is filled with highlight reels, curated moments that make other people buy into the idea that life is perfect—and if yours isn't, you're doing something wrong.

That illusion does not hold up under scrutiny. A Boston University study examining couples and social media use found that frequent posting was associated with higher levels of dissatisfaction and conflict in relationships (Valenzuela, Halpern, and Katz 2014). In other words, the couples most eager to project happiness online were often experiencing more strain behind the scenes. What looks aspirational on the surface is frequently compensatory underneath.

It just goes to show that taking advice from strangers online about your style sets you up for failure. The beauty and the sheen of it all makes you look around your perfectly *normal* life and feel like something is missing.

And shopping for clothes gives us a massive dopamine hit to counter that manufactured feeling of envy and unhappiness. But then you end up with clothes that get worn maybe once or even sit in the closet with tags still attached. Each tagged, unwashed garment is a moment of guilt each time you see it, and your closet slowly but surely gets more bloated.

Think about the last few pieces of clothing that you bought. *Why* did you buy it? Is it good quality? How many times do you expect to wear it? Are you still happy you got it, or do you already feel buyer's remorse?

There's no shame here. I occasionally still fall victim to a piece of clothing that is less than perfect. Thank goodness for generous return policies! But a Youniform requires you to slow down and be mindful about what clothes you choose to wear. You gain the ability to say no to influencer culture. Sure, you might occasionally see something and realize it actually *is* perfect for you. But the other 99% of the time, you can simply keep scrolling and know that your own sense of style is solid.

What Fashion Reveals About Our Need to Belong

"On Wednesdays we wear pink." A millennial cult classic, *Mean Girls* (2004) makes a lot of statements about high school and belonging. But this quote in particular, off the cuff and one of the "rules" of being cool, actually says a whole lot about fashion, in particular, trends and how we approach them.

If you are too busy chasing the next trend, you never have the space to figure out what you really love.

Maybe you think that you're not into trends, and you never fall victim to trending fashion styles. But the truth is that we all do, even if it's a subtle shift. For over a decade, skinny jeans were *it*. I vividly remember when they first became a thing.

In my circles, it was the male worship pastors at church wearing them with plaid flannel in the hipster vibe, becoming the subject of endless memes. I thought it was weird and clung to my bootcut jeans. But as time goes by, what once seemed unusual feels normal. We see it everywhere, so it becomes accepted rather than trending. The same happened when skinny jeans suddenly went *out* of fashion several years ago, thanks to the younger generations refusing to be so constrained.

Millennial moms took to social media, posting that you could pry their skinny jeans out of their cold, dead hands. They would *never* wear wide legs again. But, as always, people became desensitized, and wide-leg pants are now the majority. And when you read this book, we may have swung back in the other direction yet again, but that doesn't matter—because your Youniform is *your* timeless staple and you don't have to worry about trends coming and going.

These wild types of clothing preference shifts used to be generational, and a 20-year cycle was to be expected. Just as you are reaching middle age, the teenagers adopt the style of your youth (and yes, it's sometimes horrifying). The rise of fast fashion has of course sped this up and also made the distinctions less obvious. Some shifts are more widespread and long-lasting (like jean silhouette), while others are a flash bang that comes and goes faster than you can pay off the credit card bill (like socks with sandals). We could rehash the issues with cheap clothes, but following trends without understanding yourself leads to a loss of style—your own style.

At the heart of our desire to own trending things is the basic desire to fit in. Abraham Maslow designed a pyramid that represents how humans seek to fulfill their needs. You may have heard of it: Maslow's Hierarchy of Needs.

Belonging is right in the middle, above basic needs and security, but below esteem and self-actualization. Fitting in and belonging is our basic human desire to be accepted and loved by other people.

We rarely realize that how we dress is 100% related to that aspect of life. Over the years I have heard hundreds of women say they want other people to tell them, "You look so put together." They want their husbands to notice them; they don't want to look over *or* underdressed; they choose clothes to impress other women, and on and on...

So we end up wearing pink on Wednesdays because our friends are doing it, even if we hate the color. Obviously, this is satire, but how often have you worn clothes you didn't really like just because everyone else was doing it? I'll bet more than once.

Cue the mantra "If all your friends jumped off a bridge..." They taught you a hundred ways to avoid peer pressure when you were younger, but when it comes to clothes, somehow it doesn't stick. But what if being stylish had nothing to do with trends, and everything to do with being true to yourself?

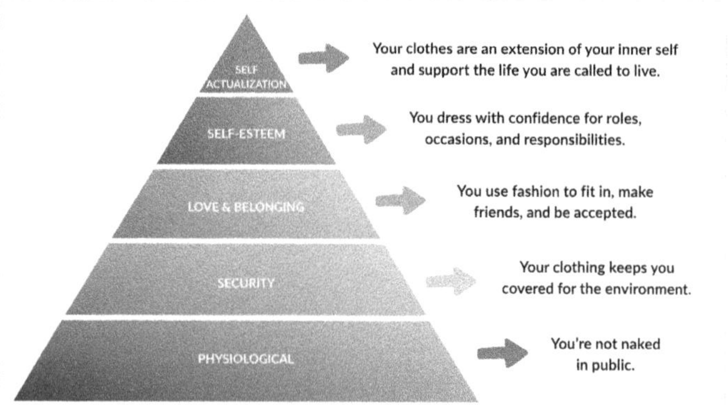

Figure 3.1 Personal style hierarchy based on Maslow's Hierarchy of Needs (for full color images visit youniformbook.com)

When we consider Maslow's Hierarchy of Needs through the lens of fashion, we can see what drives the purchases we make, and what steps we can take to go to the next level.

Our physiological needs deal with having clothing, period. Our basic need is to be dressed in public, and clothing is considered in this category on the overall spectrum. I assume that if you're reading this book, you are not here.

Security needs encompass clothing our body for the immediate weather needs around us. If you live in a cold climate, you have an adequate coat, gloves, hat, and shoes to keep you warm. Here is where budgetary considerations come into play in the fashion hierarchy. If you can meet the basic needs to be healthy in your clothes, you are not here.

Love and belonging are where trends lie. This is where most women live their lives, consuming fashion. Many of the things discussed in this book, from fast fashion to shopping hauls, deal with trying to fit in through clothing choice.

The line into esteem is a bit blurry, because many of the needs for love and belonging also fit in here. But this is where we break out into how we dress for different occasions. Having a wide and varied wardrobe that works for career interviews, funerals, and even confidently choosing a Mother of the Bride dress fits into this category.

Finally, we have self-actualization, and this is where I want to take you.

All the other needs have to be met first: financial, security, belonging, esteem, before you can express yourself fully through style.

But if you are too busy chasing the next trend to fit in, then you never have the space to figure out what you really love.

Take a long hard look at your relationship to style trends. Do you watch them carefully, always ready to try the next thing? Is it because if you were to stop and think for a minute, you'd be uncomfortable thinking about what you actually like? How often do you feel buyer's remorse, regretting a purchase almost instantly, or frequently returning purchases? Does your closet contain tagged items you've never worn that are trends? Do you remember why at that moment you bought it?

I'm not suggesting to never buy anything trendy; by all means, if it's 100% love, go for it. But instead of a trendy style, consider creating your own timeless style. One that grows with you, that is so beautiful for you that no one notices if you're wearing skinny jeans in a wide-leg world, because you look so stunning that no one cares.

The Real Reason You Wear the Same Things

I have a favorite spatula for cooking scrambled eggs, and I have a different favorite for cooking meat. Sometimes my oldest uses the meat spatula for the eggs, and it drives me nuts. If I use it for breakfast, I have to wash it before cooking dinner. I also have three potato peelers, but I will only use one of them, because the others feel funny in my grip. And yes, perhaps I'm overly obsessive with a few sensory issues, but the fact remains that we have favorites in an endless number of categories. I'd bet you have a favorite spot on the sofa, a favorite place to get coffee, and definitely a favorite pair of jeans.

I used to have a favorite pair of jeans. Disclaimer: I have always been a Youniform shopper; *if you love it buy it again* has been my motto for over a decade. My favorite pair of jeans were the Old Navy super skinny jeggings. And even though I bought several pairs in the space of a few months, there was one pair that was just better than the rest. And when they were dirty, I was always slightly annoyed that I had to wear another pair, because the length was longer and they were a bit tighter in the waist. But that one pair of jeans...perfection.

At the beginning of this book, I shared some statistics with you, one of which was the fact that for most women, only 10% of their wardrobe is actually being worn. When you break down the numbers for that fact, if the average woman owns 150 items of clothing, that means she's regularly rotating through fifteen items. Which is a shockingly small amount for most people to consider. But think about what that probably includes...jeans, shirts, some cardigans or jackets, maybe a dress. And what of the other 90%? Hanging idly in the closet, occasionally pulled out to wear, but usually relegated back to oblivion because something about that piece just feels *wrong*.

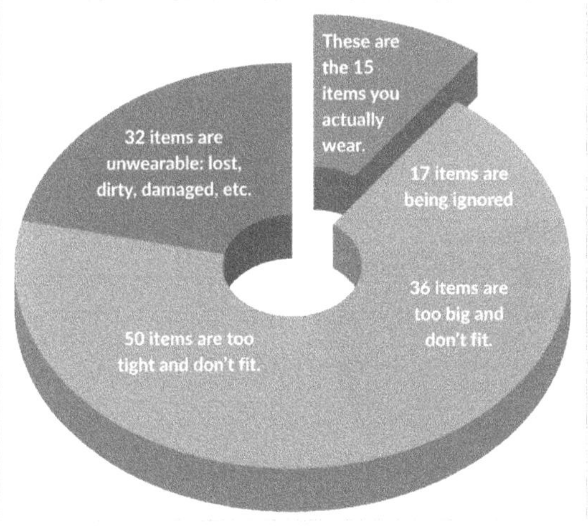

Figure 3.2 Breakdown of 150 items of clothing based on average closet usage statistics.

I'd like to challenge you to flip that statistic upside down. What if you wore even 80% of your closet regularly, and the other 20% was unworn and ignored? You now have over 100 pieces of clothing to wear. Which suddenly seems like an awful lot of options compared to fifteen. Especially when you realize you are pretty happy with those fifteen, since they are your favorites.

Imagine instead that you had about fifty items of clothing that you actually loved and enjoyed wearing. Each pair of jeans was your favorite, and each shirt was a favorite. You had clothes for work and clothes for play and clothes for rain or shine. Every day, getting dressed was like meeting your closest friends for brunch, because your clothing actually brought you joy and reflected the real you.

I want you to go into your closet and find your favorite piece of clothing. Put it on and look at yourself in the mirror. Enjoy the memories that item brings up of the times you wore it and were happy. Think about how, when, and why you purchased that one item. Clearly state three words that describe how it makes you feel.

Take that level of style contentment and multiply it times every piece.

That is what you can unlock when you adopt Youniform dressing for every part of your life. It's a beautiful thing to walk in your closet and feel good about what you own, get excited about getting dressed in clothes that fit your life and style, and walk out confident each day in your favorite things.

Why Most Women Never Claim Their Style

I'll never forget the day I told my business coach, "I want to inspire women to throw off the expectations about what they should wear and embrace being unique."

She got this uncomfortable look on her face and said, "Most people aren't ready to hear that."

But I think we have to lean into the part that makes us uncomfortable to come out on the other side as confident women.

I hated junior high school. My daughter asked me the other day if I would want to be her age again (11) and I sharply replied "Heck no, there isn't enough money in the world for me to relive ages thirteen to twenty-five." I made a lot of mistakes (those would need their own book to be frank) but I was a victim of bullying in grades 8-9. It's funny in retrospect, because I begged my mom to buy me the trendy brand-name jeans, but it didn't actually make me fit in. I wanted so badly to be part of the cool kids, which is a common thread for many teenagers.

That's why they make so many questionable choices, under the guise of "but all my friends are doing it." I like to think that we all eventually grow out of that phase, and reach that old lady space of not giving a flip what anyone thinks. But for some, I think it never really goes away, and I find that to be a sad prison to keep ourselves in.

Dare to be unique. Be yourself. Wear whatever brings you joy. Don't let the culture tell you who to be or what to wear.

I remember my grandmother enjoyed shopping and clothes. My mom didn't really, and I bet my early love for clothing came from my grandma. One day when she was over ninety, I realized that she had stopped caring so much about what she wore, favoring "old lady" elastic waist pants and elderly woman shirts. But then she broke her hip and rallied through the surgery. Afterwards, one leg was several inches shorter than the other, and she had to wear special shoes with lifts (that were admittedly kinda ugly). My mom told me about the day she started crying in the car over her shoes, saying, "What have I become?" I think this story illustrates that there's always a piece of us that cares what other people will think. And even in her twilight years, there was still something that could shake the confidence she had rightly earned over nine decades.

The majority of my most transformative clients are circling menopause. I used to wonder why that was until I started feeling the effects of perimenopause and went down the research rabbit trail. Several influential women in this space made a similar statement about how menopause can be incredibly freeing for many women, because it's a time when they focus on what brings them joy. They are freed from the societal expectations of being young, or being a mom, and can make decisions about life based on wisdom. I realized that the reason these clients come to me is that I am quietly saying the thing that shall not be named...

Dare to be unique. Be yourself. Wear whatever brings you joy. Don't let the culture tell you who to be or what to wear.

And that message is controversial.

Because we long to fit in, to be non-disruptive, to be acceptable to society. But our inner self fights to be free.

Embracing your own sense of signature style can set you free. It can embolden you to become the fierce, confident version of yourself that deserves a place at the table. It can open doors that were closed, because you command the room in a way that you did not before. It can set you on a path to accomplish things you only dreamed of (like writing a book). When you align the inner woman with the outer presentation, you become a force of nature in the lives of those around you.

Studies have noted that individuals with higher self-confidence have more success in all areas of their life (XAP Corporation 2024). Although the chicken and egg conundrum remains as to which comes first, they note that the increased confidence is often a result of self-efficacy, or the belief that you can accomplish something. I know that one small win often leads to bigger wins as your confidence in any area grows.

So, think about your expression of style as the testing ground for your confidence. The journey of style is a personal development transformation, and as such, requires steps and success along a pathway. I'm excited to show you the whole path in the coming chapters, but I want you to understand that each small win builds. Every time you put on an outfit and get a compliment, it reinforces that the process is working. When you can say *no* to the cutest pair of shoes because you recognize that they aren't really your style, you begin to believe in yourself. You move from "I can do this," to "I *am* doing this, and it feels great."

And when you feel great, you look great.

You can't fake confidence. Look at a candid group of women out having fun and study each woman individually. You'll see some of them with shoulders back, big smiles, but others are shrinking in and making themselves smaller. Often, it's not the prettiest girl that looks the most confident, but her confidence makes her stand out more than the rest.

Self-confidence will always be your most attractive asset. In the rest of this book, I'm going to share my style secrets with you, including the framework to build repeatable outfits using personal Youniforms. Each step is more than checking a box or following directions. It's about digging deep to find the person you were created to be. To unleash your potential and desires, to show up boldly and live a life of purpose. Some tasks will seem hard, and those are the ones that will set you free the most.

You do not have to keep believing that style belongs to other people. It is not reserved for the fashionable, the thin, or the naturally confident. It is something you can understand, practice, and claim. And I want you to remember this one thing as we move on...

Don't be afraid to stand out. Nothing great was ever accomplished by being invisible.

Chapter Three Highlights

- The Spotlight Effect convinces us that others closely notice our outfits, when in reality they rarely do.
- Trend cycles and influencer culture capitalize on our desire to belong, encouraging consumption over discernment.
- Reaching for the same clothes repeatedly is not a failure of creativity but a signal of alignment and comfort.
- Lasting style confidence emerges only after basic needs are met and comparison no longer dictates decisions.
- A Youniform replaces trend chasing with cohesion, allowing personal style to reflect identity rather than insecurity

Part Two

The Youniform System

"I love having a Youniform for every part of my life! I commute over an hour each way to work, so I need outfits I can grab quickly without overthinking. Stacey's Youniform system makes getting dressed effortless—I have go-to silhouettes that work for every occasion. My favorite pants style looks just as good as dress pants, jeans, or loungewear, all while staying true to my style goals.

"I used to think you shouldn't buy the same top in every color, but Stacey showed me that when you find a silhouette you love, you absolutely can —as long as the colors fit your palette!"

Melinda

Four

The Five Stages of Style

"You should start a blog about it."

I could never have imagined the outcome those words would have on me. How a challenge to share what I was discovering would become a global business helping others.

My one dress was serving me well, and I was proving all the internet gurus wrong. I craved a capsule wardrobe, so I spent a month searching online for tips on making one with dresses, but I only found articles that talked about the advantages of separate pieces.

Most capsule wardrobe examples feature a variety of pieces and display a distinct classic aesthetic. That's where most systems fail. Instead of assuming that one formula fits every woman, Youniform begins with you—your lifestyle, your body, and your purpose—so every outfit serves your real life, not an idealized version of it. Wardrobe essential lists cater to a specific minimalist style and contain things like jeans, a black blazer, white button-down shirts, and a little black dress. But that's not me, and that kind of wardrobe alone made me feel unhappy and bored.

I even began researching skirt capsule wardrobes to see if the answer was hiding there, but they still featured one or two dresses in the whole mix. I admit I let this go to my head a bit and started trying to fit my desires into all the frameworks online.

I got lost and started adding various items that were considered "essential", and my one-dress concept fell apart. But I was unhappy, and life got more complicated with each closet addition. I started trying to use separates again, but this time hacked to just skirts. Believing I needed more variety to have a functional wardrobe, I tried to collect wardrobe essentials by substituting unique pieces. I bought a pencil skirt and liked it, so I bought five more. Then I tried a circle skirt and liked it, so I bought five more of those too.

But in reality? I wasn't wearing any of them. Every morning I'd open the drawer and feel frustrated, staring at skirts piled so high the drawer wouldn't close. They were overflowing, a reminder of all the wrong turns I'd taken. I'd stand there wondering if something was wrong with me. Why couldn't I just stick to a simple plan? Why did I have to keep overcomplicating my style that used to feel so easy? My stomach would twist into knots as that old voice whispered that I would never figure this out.

As I tried all these closet experiments, it became clear how much I didn't know about style. Maybe you've had the same realization—that getting dressed out of habit means you rarely stop to think about your actual style preferences. Traditional style advice teaches variety without a strategy. The Youniform Framework reverses this by creating repeatable combinations that work every time, so you never waste money chasing pieces that don't actually fit your life.

The reason we like one shirt over another all boils down to intricate style theories, and learning those - well, that took me some time. But it turned out that I could define my style following proven principles, and you can too. Your style preference could be as simple as preferring one type of neckline over another. Without you realizing it, your eyes notice things your brain doesn't label, like body shape, height, and if your features are rounded or angular, which all affect what looks good on you, even down to the best necklines.

Learning these nuances changed the game for me. They helped me finally let go of everything that didn't fit who I was and focus only on what I truly loved.

Over time, I saw clear patterns emerge. Again and again, clients told me they didn't know how to put outfits together. Every time, the root cause traced back to the same thing: not understanding their body harmony. Once they learned it, everything clicked. Outfits started making sense. Confidence followed.

As my closet bloated with all those unworn skirts I tried to make work, I had to stop and ask where one should even start in this process. I began experimenting with different style ideas, devouring books and reading blogs, combing discussion boards and exploring how we use style as personal expression.

That led to the realization that personal style is a *journey*.

When we're children, we inherit the style of our parents' choices. When we're teens and young adults, it's all about experimentation and pushing the boundaries. In our twenties and thirties, we settle into the style of those around us and adopt what many would consider mainstream style.

Then as we creep towards forty, gravity, perimenopause, and a host of challenges stop us in our tracks. We wrestle with the concept of how we look as time marches on, and we feel out of touch. If you're GenX or Millennial, you likely know exactly what

I mean. In our twenties, we don't care about style tricks and hacks, because we're having fun and everything looks good on us. But as we get older, we have more insight, wisdom, intuition, and often more money to invest in *looks maxxing* (a newfangled way of saying "dressing to look your best").

Most of my clients come to me near this age milestone, triggered not just by the physical changes, but by a deep realization that it's time to be who they *truly* are. No more masks, no more pretending, just full authenticity.

But there's power in this place, as you now get the privilege of deciding who you want to be for the second half of your life. And even as your personal journey of getting dressed shifts with each decade, the journey to finding authentic style is an ongoing process.

It's easy to think that finding your unique style is a one-time process, but you are always changing, and your style needs to evolve with you. This doesn't require a reinvention of your entire closet, though; instead, it asks you to use a magnifying glass and start with the big picture to refine more with each pass.

It's this process that you will learn here: the Five Stages of Style. You will uncover the cycle of personal style exploration and see how you dance between each stage, making small tweaks as you change. This framework will help you recognize where you are right now and what comes next, so you can stop guessing and start building a style that truly fits who you are.

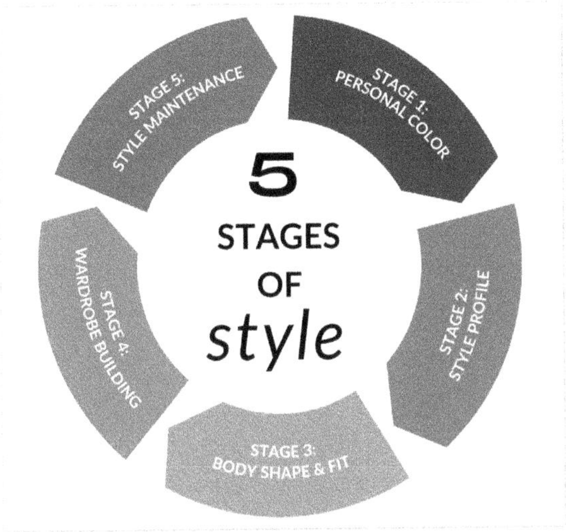

Figure 4.1 The Five Stages of Style showing the circular process of refining personal style and the closet (for full color images visit youniformbook.com)

By the end of this chapter, you'll know exactly which of the five stages you're in right now, and more importantly, you'll have the roadmap to move confidently into the next phase of your style evolution.

When I started writing the blog back in 2020, I asked myself where to begin. The massive wins I had experienced with *personal color* made it the perfect place to build a foundation. This is where your style journey starts, with a powerful tool that lasts a lifetime.

Finding your best colors leads to creating your *style profile* and expressing it with your wardrobe. This brings your outer style into alignment with the inner you, as the clothes mirror who you are without effort.

With these two tactics, you've already increased your confidence and made friends with the woman in the mirror. Discovering *body shape and fit* is the next step. Instead of thinking about the shape of fruits or hourglasses, you get to examine the flesh and bones of your body through the lens of inheritance. You'll understand that the planes of your face and curve (or lack thereof) in your body are simply a reflection of your genetics. The body you've got—from your parents, grandparents, and beyond—is the body we're dressing, and you'll finally see why some clothes just don't work for you.

With all of this foundational knowledge about how you are created uniquely beautiful, it's time to start mindfully curating your closet. In *wardrobe building* you will apply the Youniform framework to every part of your closet. This means the days of impulse buys are over, as you will discover a revolutionary plan for curating a closet based on go-to outfits.

This is the meat of building a closet you love, and this is the time to reflect on every item you have. With beautiful clothes, newfound confidence, and mindful intention, you enter the *style maintenance* phase of your journey. High-level strategies for shopping, regular editing and decluttering, and image freedom become your focus.

Imagine walking past the mirror every day and not obsessing over every tiny flaw, but instead moving on with your day knowing you are dressed just right. You no longer let your appearance control your self-worth, recognizing it's just a neutral aspect of your life.

When you're no longer consumed by how you look (because you're stunning!) your energy is now free to experience your life. Being your genuine self daily leads to clearer goals, better relationships, and more meaningful conversations.

Your closet is no longer stealing your joy, but a place that launches you into the richness of your life. Your clothing is a tool, and your style is now a part of who you are. And as time changes you, your foundation is solid to *revisit the journey, making small renovations* along the way.

The Cool Closet Reset that Builds Your Confidence

I love to start any style transformation with a powerful process of gaining clarity about using color. I've found that doing this one thing will upgrade any closet by around fifty percent. The improvement comes from several things: getting rid of unflattering items (10%), reduced shopping mistakes (10%), and the confidence that comes from wearing your best colors (30%). When you use color as an organizational framework, it creates beauty out of chaos.

After hundreds of transformations, I've noticed a common thread. Many women start their color journey just for fun: maybe they saw color analysis online or remembered their mom having it done back in the eighties. But suddenly, something shifts. They understand the focus is not merely colors or clothing. They finally see the women they were always meant to be, rediscovering themselves in the process.

Personal color refers to the process of building your closet based on the strategy of color analysis, which we'll discuss in depth later in this book. I discovered this method by chance when I was feeling lost and trying to make sense of different styles. It turns out I wasn't reinventing the wheel. Stylists and designers have been using color as the foundation for decades; I had just found my way to it.

My early posts on Radiantly Dressed—which are still very popular—explain the twelve color types and how they can help you look better, create a capsule wardrobe, and improve your style. The first service I launched involved performing virtual color analysis, and color reports remain a core offer.

And I have seen the value and impact play out time and time again. You could solve half of your style problems just by making this one change. Many women frequently halt their journey here, finding that the confidence and clarity through color is enough for them. But I am going to push you to keep going, letting this first step be a huge win and the impetus to continue to create your true signature style. Commit to a full transformation and continue your journey after you first discover your colors and see your natural beauty.

When we use color to create limits in our closet, it makes getting dressed easier. This is because it helps you organize things, makes buying and getting rid of things clear, and helps you pick outfits.

Designing the perfect closet is a billion-dollar industry ("US Home Organizers and Storage Market Size & Share Analysis - Industry Research Report - Growth Trends," n.d.). The fact of the matter is that Americans simply have too much stuff, and businesses jumped happily into the gap to provide solutions to the problem. I remember when I was younger and money was tight, walking through the Container Store felt like stepping into a dream of perfect order. I couldn't afford any of it then, so I found creative ways to organize using budget-friendly finds from Walmart and the Dollar Store.

Regarding closets, designing the perfectly curated walk-in mini store has become an object of aspiration. From hanging bar placement to elaborate, lighted shoe shelving, built-in dresser drawers and gracefully dangling chandeliers, the celebrity-style closet at home can be lovely.

But we can create beauty in our closet organization even if you have a tiny two-foot-deep version with builder basic bars and those annoying half shelves. And we do it by using color to create a stunning display of your personal inventory. Even the clothes we don't love so much become more beautiful when they're arranged in a gradient of hues.

You can now see what you have, whether it's fifty black shirts (I see you), or loads of yellow and reds but no blues. The visual presentation gives us clarity about what we currently have, and we can use that to manage the inventory of our clothes.

Back to the Container Store: I don't know if you've ever worked retail, but a few times a year companies perform inventory on what's in stock in their store. They use this system to catalog and reconcile what they ordered versus what is on the shelf to find and prevent losses.

This process was always annoying and entertaining to me, watching a dozen contractors come in with fancy inventory machines tacked to their belts, climbing shelves and scanning away like robots, highly focused on the task at hand. I'm not saying you need a complex system like that for your closet, but it's good to know what clothes you have to keep track of them.

Two processes are a regular part of that cycle: shopping and decluttering. A color system gives you a base system for making those decisions. While shopping, consider whether you need another black shirt when you already have a dozen, or if a different color might be a better choice. For decluttering, you can use personal color knowledge to provide a boundary for what you will keep. Discovered you don't like emerald green and never reach for it? Let it go and make room for clothing that you will actually wear.

But the biggest gain from using personal color to design our closets is the ease of choosing outfits. When we can see everything we have displayed in a color-coded arrangement, our choices become clearer.

Many people admit to dopamine dressing, or choosing clothes based on how they feel and improving that state. Often that means choosing one item to start your daily outfit and using it as inspiration. For this example, let's assume you have a printed skirt with a black background and florals in shades of pink, yellow, and white. You might be inclined to choose the shirt you wore last time, but using a color system, you can easily look at your tops, see several options for each of the skirt's colors, and select one based on interest and joy.

Color in our closet provides stability, organization, and helps us make easier decisions. Organize your clothes by color using this system, and see if it improves your wardrobe, even if you don't know much about colors.

First, you will need to sort your items into four categories: tops, bottoms, completer pieces (blazers, cardigans, jackets, etc.), and one-piece outfits like jumpsuits and dresses. Each group forms its own section to be sorted by color. Don't get hung up here worrying about sorting by length or any other measure; we are going to let color lead the way.

The basic premise of a Color Coded Closet uses this order, but I will give more details below. From left to right, the order is white, silver, beige, yellow, orange, red, pink, purple, blue, teal, green, brown, gray, and black. This follows a general progression from light to dark, using the relationship of colors on the Munsell color wheel to bridge the gap. But since colors are nuanced, I'd like to provide a few nuggets and hints.

Figure 4.2 Color Coded Closet color system to organize your closet from light neutrals to dark neutrals through the rainbow.

White refers to true white and anything that is near white, like ivory or cream. The following two colors of silver and beige typically refer to light colored neutrals, and you will have to use your own perception to decide at which point a gray shirt belongs in silver at the front or gray at the back. Each of the four sections should have a bookend of light neutral on the left and dark neutral on the right, and they mirror each other.

I love clarity out of chaos! Moving into the color section, we start with yellow because it's the lightest option and let it carry us around the color wheel. Some colors form a bridge, like pink spanning red and purple, and teal spanning blue and green. It's worth noting here that some people have a very acute eye for color variations, while others do not. If you struggle to see colors clearly and distinctly, don't get caught up here in perfection. Do the best you can and know that your Color Coded Closet is going to be a vast improvement from before.

Now it's time for you to do this process; start with your tops, move to bottoms, do the fun completer pieces next, and your one-piece items last. Start with your light neutrals, go through the colors, and finish with dark neutrals. When you are done, step back and admire your work. Make note of any color schemes you see emerging from your newly organized closet and what that might say about your personal preferences. And know that later we are going to go very deep in this area. We aren't done yet!

Your journey through personal color has just begun, and this will be a profound foundational piece for you in this process. Take the powerful win, make the first step by creating your color-organized closet, and let it simplify and provide clarity in your closet.

Create Clarity in 30 Minutes with the Style Goals Exercise

Color gives us a powerful perspective on our clothing, but it also illustrates the impact of our style on how we communicate. We can easily use color to affect our mood and interaction with the world. From black at funerals to red as a power color, what we're wearing is a form of nonverbal communication.

As a lost twenty-something college dropout, I could never decide what I wanted to be when I grew up. I changed my major about a dozen times in community college before finally quitting because I was completely out of control. When the opportunity to finish came to me at twenty-five, my slightly more mature self jumped at the chance to achieve this "required" milestone (if you know, you know).

Still completely clueless about my life path, I chose communication as my major with psychology as my minor (I started with economics as a minor, but one hard-to-understand professor killed it for me). And I finished in two years, leaving with a diploma that said, "B.S. in Business Communication." It's a soft degree, and I took courses on things like small group dynamics, interpersonal communication, and public relations.

I find it funny that what I have often considered being comparable to a degree in underwater basket weaving now has a place here inside my work on style. Little did I know that this 'soft' degree would become the foundation for understanding how style functions as powerful nonverbal communication in my work with hundreds of professional women.

Every day we are communicating something about ourselves by the clothing on our body.

Communication is defined as "a process by which information is exchanged between individuals through a common system of symbols, signs, or behavior" (Merriam Webster 2025). We know words are verbal communication and body language is nonverbal communication. But our clothing also becomes a powerful method of communication as all three: symbols, signs, and behaviors.

Think back to your teen years to see this in action. For many people, this is a time of high exploration with style, also wound up in rebellion and finding our place in the hierarchy of young adulthood. At my high school, groups and cliques broke off into small sets, becoming almost gang-like in their territorial nature over who took what position in the courtyard. But beyond their shared experiences at that point in life, their clothing choices showed which group they belonged to.

The preppy kids who lived in the fancy neighborhoods wore the expensive brands (I won't date myself, but brown leather loafers were so in). Goth kids wore all black, white-out makeup, and had silver chains hanging here and there. The jocks with their jerseys on Friday or the kids with their secondhand clothes.

The clothing styles marked high school society and communicated a message of "you belong with us" or "get out." And if you dared to embrace a style that wasn't in your clique, the harassment would begin from all sides. As an adult, I now understand the value of traditional school uniforms in the learning process, and realizing this played a part in the lightbulb moment that led to Youniform. School uniforms work because they remove an element of social class, allowing students to focus on gaining knowledge. Style Youniforms work for the same reason: they remove cultural comparison so adults can focus on living with purpose. Our clothing speaks volumes about who we are, what we're doing, where we are trying to belong, and even what kind of day we are having.

If you are giving an important presentation, you want your clothing to express that you are confident and capable. While a power color like red might be your first thought, you opt instead for a well-fitting ensemble in a trustworthy navy, its clean lines and stellar fit indicating that you care about your appearance. For a bit of a bolster, you might choose undergarments with structure to remind you to stand up straight and look the part. And you can finish with heels, because the elevation gives you a different perspective and makes you feel powerful.

Conversely, if you have a migraine, suits and high heels are the last thing on your mind. You desire comfort and coziness, opting for pants with some stretch, your favorite sweater, and a blanket to give a feeling of security. And while you're probably not having guests when you feel unwell, your clothing is still communicating that you aren't at your best and need some additional TLC.

Everyday we make a choice about what to wear. Every day we are communicating something about ourselves by the clothing on our body. So let's be intentional with the message we're sending.

Most people do this without realizing they're sending mixed messages through their clothes. The Youniform Framework eliminates that confusion by aligning your wardrobe with your message, so what you wear always reflects who you truly are.

An exercise I do with my clients to get clarity on their personal style communication is called Style Goals. These are three powerful words that form a baseline for what you want to say to the world through clothing. You can use these words daily to check if what you're wearing will have the intended effect of telling people who you are and what your values are.

Yes, our clothing can really do all that!

First, let me walk you through the process of developing your three words, and then I'll provide some insight about how to structure them. This exercise takes about 30 minutes but creates clarity that will serve you for years.

You'll need to find a place where you can think and focus, because we're going to do some deep exploration and begin with a brain dump. I always recommend paper for this part, as studies show that our brains remember things better when we write them down (Van der Weel and Van der Meer 2024).

As with any brainstorming exercise, please don't edit. Write everything, even if it seems ridiculous or foolish or nonsensical. Let your pen have free reign to dream up all the possibilities that could exist for your style; we will edit them shortly.

These questions make you think about how you want the world to see you, so we can tap into themes that occur. These themes are your inner self, and this is who we want to share with the world, without saying a word. We want our clothes and style to embody our truest inner self, so that we become authentically aligned with every interaction and moment. Begin with these questions and write as much as you can that comes to mind:

1. What are the values that matter most to you, and that you want to express to the world?

2. What emotions do you want to feel, and what feelings do you want to inspire in others?

3. What are the rich inner parts of yourself that you want to share?

Imagine your personal style at its aspirational best...describe this style with no limitations.

Now it's time to find order in the chaos of ideas that you just generated. Go back through all the words and phrases you just brainstormed and look for recurring themes. Group them into similar buckets, ideally aiming for three distinct sections that overlap. You will start to see words or phrases that stand out and resonate; highlight or circle those in each of your three buckets.

Finally, the hardest part, choosing a single word for each of your idea sets. Most of my clients struggle with this step, so I want to encourage you to keep going. The first pass doesn't have to be perfect, but finishing will give you profound insight. For each of the three buckets or idea sets you've collected, I want you to pick just *one. word.*

Your word should be conceptual in nature and encompass the general theme of the collection of words and phrases. Don't worry about the dictionary definition of the word or any connotations. Focus only on what the word means *to you*. It's your style goal and no one else's. Even if someone else were to choose the same word, the depth and richness of meaning is unique to each of you.

Repeat this process until you have three distinct words that encompass the style you aspire to and how you want to present yourself to the world. Then, for each word, write your own definition, including what it means to you in the context of your personal style. To provide an illustration, I asked my clients to share some of their own, and here are just a few examples:

Holly chose creative, feminine, and free-spirited to express her bohemian, artistic streak and desire to be modest and beautiful.

Evelyn chose feminine, light, and connected to express how she wants to be seen as someone who connects with others in an easy, gracious way.

Donna chose natural, enduring, and serene to express how she wants to appear timeless and elegantly simple in her style.

These examples show how special this process is, and how focusing on a single word to guide your style can help you choose outfits. My clients frequently share feedback after this exercise, stating how they can choose their clothes more quickly each day, shaving off five to ten minutes of the decision-making process. To complete your Style Goal creation exercise, I invite you to do a bit of reflection to double check these are aligned with who you are right now.

- Do these words both reflect who you are *and* who you want to be?
- Do these concepts cover a range of situations and interactions?
- Does it resonate at a deep level?
- Does it align with your values?

Communication is one thing that sets apart humanity and lets us build civilizations (indeed, the power of language is perfectly demonstrated in the Biblical story of Babel). Our clothing is a powerful form of nonverbal communication, and what we wear speaks volumes to those around us without ever saying a word.

Harness this power of style to make sure that you are dressing with intention every day, bringing richness to your interactions with others, expressing your excitement and willingness to do great things, and aligning function and purpose with every outfit.

This Exercise Will Transform How You See Your Body Forever

Having great colors and specific clarity makes a big difference in how we present ourselves in style, but at some point, we have to address the way we actually wear the clothing. Perhaps the most difficult and frustrating part of getting dressed is choosing clothes that fit and flatter our unique body shape.

There are loads of different ways of defining body type for personal style, and we'll touch on that in a later chapter. But for now, I want to focus on the concepts of shape and silhouette to get a new perspective on making peace with our bodies.

When I mention shape, you may think naturally of things like triangles or circles, and in fashion we can use these ideas as well. When you consider clothing construction, you'll find these basic shapes make up many parts of any garment.

Pants and skirts can be made rectangular or cut more in a circle, changing the way the item looks. Necklines are either angular like V-necks (triangle) or square, or rounded like crew necks, scoop necks, or sweetheart styles. Shapes are found across all clothing types, and there's a secret here that the shapes on your body do well by matching the shapes on your clothing. For example, if your shoulders are gently rounded, curved necklines like scoop or sweetheart styles will mirror that shape beautifully. If your shoulders are straighter, angular necklines like a V or square can create better harmony.

This is a micro perspective of looking at all the individual parts of your body to find the tiny details of style that make you look your best. The macro perspective deals with the concept of silhouette.

When I was a teen, my best friend and I went to the county fair every summer. We rode questionably safe rides, ate funnel cake until we were nauseated, and spent all our allowance on silly crafts and trinkets. One of the art souvenirs that I remember well was the profile silhouette drawing, where the artist would render your facial side profile in black on a white background. I still think about this years later every time I do a consultation for a client because it was the first time I truly saw myself from the outside. I did not know what my side profile looked like until that day, and I remember being shocked by the shape of my cheeks and nose.

A body is just a body, and we deserve to feel good at every shape and size.

Silhouette is defined as "the outline or general shape of something", in this case, the female body. This is something we can create and draw to get a baseline understanding of our own personal body silhouette. This provides us with a fresh perspective on what our body requires of the clothing we put on.

I do an exercise with my clients where they outline their body while wearing tight clothes, similar to how an artist once traced my face when I was thirteen. It can be challenging mentally, but it allows them to step back and take an objective look at their body: the curves and lines and unique shapes found in all the parts. The first time I did this exercise, I was a few months postpartum with my fifth baby, and facing the reality of my current body was hard to swallow.

But a body is just a body, and we deserve to feel good at every shape and size.

My client Joanna had an amazingly beautiful realization when we were doing this exercise. A talented artist, she struggled to do this exercise because of her own body traumas, including abuse and the devastating loss of a child. But in pushing through, she ended up creating a stunning painting from the process. She realized that her silhouette was the general structure of a vase (most women are), and painted flowers spilling out of her own silhouette, representing the beauty that she held within that was waiting to burst out into the world. That realization changed everything for her. She saw her body not as something broken or limited, but as a vessel for creativity and grace. Her wardrobe shifted too, into softer fabrics, flowing lines, and colors that mirrored the warmth and light she had painted. For the first time in years, she told me she felt proud of her body, powerful and beautiful in its own way.

Now every time I see a client do this exercise, I always see a vase, full of possibility, coming in varying heights, widths, and with differing amounts of curve—each client with different flowers spilling out, making up the unique version of her. But each one is a woman filled with possibility, and the freedom in seeing yourself as simply a vessel to live richly, takes away many of those thoughts about how we "should" look.

I love these shape and silhouette exercises because they allow us to stop feeling stuck in a body that we have very little control over. If you were genetically gifted with broad shoulders, no amount of diet or exercise or even plastic surgery can change that. Accepting what *is* on our body gives us the ability to move forward and choose clothing styles that enhance our unique shape.

From micro shapes to macro silhouette, we can apply this body type awareness to choose complete outfits that match our unique vase. We can use basic tracing paper and some photos to analyze whether our clothing is working with or against our inherent shape.

Your task here is two-fold: you will create a silhouette of your body wearing form fitting clothing that does not obscure the details, and then you will create silhouette drawings wearing various outfits. You will find that the closer your outfit silhouette is to your body silhouette, the more flattering the clothing will be.

For example, if you notice your shoulders are wider than your hips, your best looks will echo that proportion. Choose structured tops or broad-shouldered bodices with little waist emphasis, paired with narrower pants or straight skirts, just like in your drawing. The goal is not to hide your shape but to mirror it, creating harmony between your body and your clothes. With hundreds of clients, I've seen the difference in confidence from choosing clothing shapes that align with their natural body design.

For the body silhouette, dress in clothing that does not obscure your shape; bathing suits or fitted bike shorts and a tank work particularly well here. You'll then take a photo of your body, at chest height, from a distance of around twelve feet away.

When you look at this picture, take a deep breath. Facing this image is often shocking for women, and they want to skip or avoid this step. But please keep pushing, because you are worth finding peace in the body that you have.

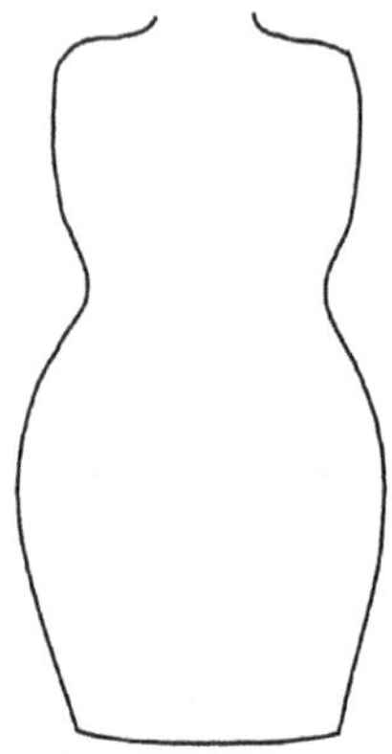

Figure 4.3 Trace your body silhouette to get an example similar to this.

With your photo in hand, you can use tracing paper and a pencil, or more advanced options like drawing software to create an outline of your body. Starting at the shoulders, trace around the edge of the shoulder line, past the bustline, coming in at the waist as needed, and continuing down past the hips to the knees. You will close the drawing at the knees and neck, forming what will appear to be a dress form—or a vase!

This is your base body silhouette.

You can use the same process to analyze various outfits in relation to your body silhouette. Choose a variety—outfits that felt great, and also those that felt off. Notice if there is a similarity or discrepancy in the silhouette of your clothes versus your body. As you refine this over time, you'll come to see the patterns of clothing that create your best fit.

When you can understand *why* certain items or outfits don't work for you, it sets you free to express your style in a way that feels perfect for you. Your confidence soars because you know you look great in your clothes and you're no longer obsessing over how you look and fidgeting with ill-fitting clothes. When we are no longer worried about ourselves, we can interact more deeply with others, focusing on them and impacting the people we care about.

Your body is a tool designed to help you live out your purpose each day, and clothing is the cultural requirement that helps you do it with confidence. Learning to embrace the shape and silhouette of the body you have allows you to accept what you have and let go of an idealized body type, because those aren't real. They leave you chasing perfection and always feeling unhappy and unfulfilled. Remember that *no body is wrong*. You were created with intention, and when you stop fighting your design, you can finally experience peace with how you look and joy in how you live.

Design Your Closet with Intention and Get Dressed in Five Minutes Flat

So far, we've covered foundation concepts about aligning your personal style with who you really are. But we've yet to talk about actually curating and planning out your closet piece by piece. This highlights why most women have clothes hanging in their closets with tags still attached—because their approach to getting dressed often starts with shopping first. It's quite common for women to have at least five items in their closet that have never been worn...at a conservative estimate of $50 per piece, that's easily $250 in wasted clothing.

The core message of this book is about building your closet using easy, repeatable outfits, which is the meat of the next several chapters. What finally helped me see the missing link was something entirely unrelated to fashion, that I discovered a hundred feet underwater.

When I was twenty-nine, I fell in love with scuba diving. It had intrigued me for over a decade when I would see it in books and movies. The idea of being in an underwater world drew me in. The first time I hopped underwater, I fell in love. It became an obsession, and I kept taking classes until I became a Divemaster—one who leads others.

Over the years, I've completed more than a hundred dives in locations around the world, but my most challenging was on the USS *Oriskany*—a sunken aircraft carrier resting 136 feet below the surface, twenty miles offshore. Down there, you're technically closer to death than life if something goes wrong. That dive taught me that preparation isn't optional.

It might seem obvious, but the tenet of every dive begins with adequate planning before entering the water. See, humans aren't made to survive underwater, and even the smallest issue can become catastrophic in a heartbeat. While fatalities are relatively rare, the most common cause is insufficient gas, which is usually a result of poor planning, or not adhering to the plan ("Scuba Diving Deaths per Year | Statistics and Causes," n.d).

My instructor used a phrase so often that it's burned into my brain "Fail to plan, and you plan to fail." I love this analogy because it's also true in wardrobe planning.

Chaos arises when we buy items here and there with no cohesive plan or guidance. However, the most functional closets emerge when we intentionally select items based on our style needs, as expressed in the first three of the Five Stages of Style. That's why my most successful clients, the ones that completely overhauled their closet into a Youniform system, all followed the step-by-step process I'm about to share with you.

Our systematic approach to wardrobe items is based on the Youniform Framework, which will be covered in great detail for much of this book. The system is based on creating repeatable outfit combinations, known as style Youniforms or a personal Youniform.

Essentially, we do the work up front in detailing specifically an outfit, including tops, bottoms, and a completer piece. Just like a basic addition problem, our three items become the Style Base that we simply duplicate.

After working with hundreds of women to create their Youniforms, I've seen how this simple three-piece formula can eliminate nearly all morning decision fatigue and bring instant clarity to getting dressed. Over 90% of my clients report getting dressed in less than five minutes after going through the program.

Armed with the knowledge from the prior style stages, you design an outfit based on small details like preferred neckline, pant leg shape, skirt cut, shirt length, and more. Our personal silhouette from stage three guides us in choosing the most flattering iteration of any outfit. This is our go-to formula, and our plan comprises buying a set number of each item for easy mix-and-match styling.

Over the years I've shared this idea with many women, and some of them naturally do this. They'll call it something like "buy it in every color." Which is a general overview, but our exploration through color in stage one gives us parameters for that as well. Every outfit combination we curated and designed thoughtfully, and we can create a style base for everything from the boardroom to the garden, based on the Youniform Framework.

For example, one of my clients created a business travel Youniform made up of several pairs of wide-leg trousers in warm autumn tones, longline vests in coral and brown polka dot, and printed button-up shirts with feminine lace details. It gave her a professional travel wardrobe that still expressed her unique personality and felt completely her.

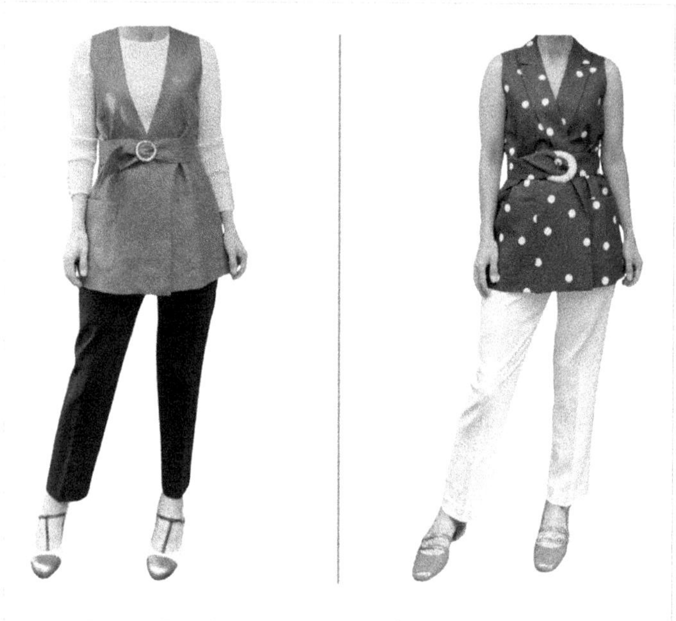

Figure 4.4 Client example showing a work Youniform with slacks and vest.

Now, instead of the closet being a place of random pieces that don't seem to work with anything else, every item has a purpose. That's not to say you can never have an outlier (a one-off item you just *love* and couldn't resist, but still make work), but these are the minority and exist because we just truly love something unique. Our wardrobe plan makes our life simpler when we get dressed and also gives us guidelines around shopping and decluttering.

The Youniform Framework provides a beautiful system for creating an entire wardrobe for your whole life. Your mornings are easy, and you can get dressed in five minutes because you have a plan for what to wear every day. Later, you will create a structure for this process to make sure everything is cohesive and functional. But before I show you the exact three-step process my clients use to identify their first Youniform, let's see what your closet is telling you right now.

1. Take a moment and do a quick inventory and answer the following questions:
2. How many items do you have with tags still attached?
3. Do you have any items that you find repeatedly hard to style, even if you genuinely like them?
4. Recall the last three purchases you made and ask yourself if you still like them enough to buy them again?
5. Identity the five items you wear the most and notice what they have in common or why you repeat them.

The Secret to Staying Effortlessly Stylish for Life

Most of my clients spend most of their time in the wardrobe planning stage, but some of them have progressed to the final style state, which finishes our chapter on this evolution. You might think that finally having the wardrobe of your dreams—which fits your life perfectly, allows you to get dressed easily, and makes you feel beautiful—is the end. But just like any process that lasts a lifetime, the ultimate step is actually ongoing maintenance.

Our lives aren't static, and even a perfectly curated closet must adapt with its owner. Throughout our lives, we go through physical changes like weight gain or getting older, lifestyle changes like starting or retiring from work, and changes in how we use our time, such as finding a new hobby. Our closet has to grow with us in all these areas and requires us to always have a hand in managing it.

Recently I polled some of my long-term clients and asked them what they were working on. One told me she was revising her color palette to reflect autumnal colors; the other said she was reworking her style goals. Another was building a style Youniform for spending more active time with grandkids, and one was still hunting for a unicorn item on her wardrobe plan. These are women who have been in my world for three to five years. They are busy women with families and established careers, yet they still find value in refining and strengthening their unique style systems. Once you learn your own Youniform, you won't stay in "figure-it-out" mode forever. You'll know what works, and adapting it as your life changes will feel easy and natural, not like starting over.

All of them have a closet they love that makes getting dressed easy. They are leaders in our community and routinely share daily-inspiration outfits. They are in tune with their personal style, and it shows. But each of them understands that this is a lifelong journey of self-discovery.

There are four main areas involved in this process, and they include shopping, decluttering, style profile revisions, and mindset work.

None of these are specific to the final stage and occur at all points of the process. But with the amount of application needed at each developmental stage, they get pushed to the side for later. However, once your immediate problem of what to wear is no longer a struggle, you can dive deeper into becoming an expert curator of personal fashion.

You will of course do some shopping throughout this process, at times in large doses as you commit to a specific Youniform, but it won't break your budget. You will still add items you need or love, but you will become a connoisseur of your style. You'll find brands you love enough to marry, use your budget to invest in quality over quantity, and create a master list for filling holes and dreaming of unicorn pieces.

Decluttering allows us to make room for what isn't serving us, making space for our well-loved clothes to breathe and be seen. Usually stage one (personal color) includes a large decluttering session as you let go of colors that don't flatter. But since no one is perfect and we all fall victim to the occasional impulse buy, intentional decluttering sessions prevent closet bloat. Clothes decluttering can truthfully be a stage zero experience, and that's why we host a group decluttering challenge every January. This is where we meet many new clients each year on their journey to a style revolution. Consider joining us next year if you want support to start fresh in your closet.

These two areas deal with the incoming and outgoing aspects of clothing inventory management. These are the tactical, tangible activities that we use to keep our closets aligned with the person we are right now. But there are internal developments that must also be addressed in the final style stage.

Our work in the first two stages of personal color and style profile are areas to revisit at least annually. We want to be sure that our style is an authentic expression of who we are right now. Perhaps our color preferences have changed, and we've noticed we're not wearing red anymore, but we have fallen in love with pink. Or maybe one of our style goals doesn't feel aligned after kids leave the nest, so we make a tweak to our words.

Living means we have the luxury of growing as a person, adapting to our purpose in new ways. Our closet should keep up with these regular audits of our personal style. We get to let go of past versions of ourselves that we have outgrown, and our clothes should reflect this forward momentum.

The final act in the stage of ongoing maintenance includes mindset work. I'm going to be honest; I used to cringe when someone said the word "mindset." To me, it was a dirty word connected to woo self-help advice and people who didn't feel confident in life. I have since revised my perspective because I need mindset work constantly; refusing this process means I stay stuck as a person. And stuck means I'm not living out the potential of my life.

I have found that mindset gremlins usually creep in heavily around stage three when we take an unfiltered look at our bodies and face the genetics of our shapes. This process of uncovering authentic style forces us to take a literal *and* figurative look in the mirror, and we rarely like what we find. Our sense of self-image is tied into the experiences of our entire lives, both good and bad.

Sometimes in the rapid pace of discovery and problem solving, we push those to the side for "later."

Later is now *here*.

It's time to do the deep work and face those monsters related to body image, sense of self, purpose, heart work, forgiveness, and acceptance. While I am not a mental health expert (and always recommend tackling these major issues with your own therapist), I have noticed a profound sense of growth and self-awareness at the "end" of this process.

As my client Lana said, "It's like my whole life finally made sense when it came to my style ... [I got to] dig deep to understand my style, who I am, who I was made to be, and what I want to reflect to the outside world. Stacey really introduced me to myself. In every area of my life, I have the confidence to show up more as myself."

The goal of building Youniforms for your life means that you get to focus on being your best self in every environment. You put in the work up front to identify your unique and intrinsic style, plan and curate outfits, and create a systemized style. By doing this, you'll embark on a journey of self-discovery, allowing you to focus less on your appearance and others' opinions, and more on living a purposeful life. Every interaction is more meaningful, and every perfectly timed encounter is a moment of focus on the other person.

As we close out this chapter on the journey of personal style expressed as five style stages, I invite you to create your own affirmation for walking this path. Use the template below and edit it for your unique voice. Write it down to bridge thought and action, and place it somewhere you can see it every day.

I commit to taking the [journey/adventure/] into personal style. I want people to see me as a [insert three style goals] woman. I desire to make an impact by [how to influence in a positive, meaningful way]. I am ready to greet the woman in the mirror with a smile every day, confident and aligned with the beauty, strength, and purpose that already exists within me.

This is why the Youniform process stands apart, because it's not about fashion at all. It's about freedom. When your wardrobe finally supports who you are, you stop striving and start living. In the next chapter, we'll dive deep into creating your very first Youniform, the one great outfit that will change how you think about getting dressed forever.

Chapter Four Highlights

- Personal style is a lifelong process that must evolve as your body, lifestyle, and purpose change.
- Most wardrobe frustration comes from skipping foundational clarity and trying to fix style problems through shopping alone.
- The Five Stages of Style provide a clear, repeatable roadmap that replaces guesswork with intention.
- Personal color is the fastest way to bring order, confidence, and simplicity to a chaotic closet.
- Clothing functions as nonverbal communication, quietly expressing who you are, what you value, and how you want to be perceived.
- Understanding body shape and silhouette removes shame and allows clothing to work in harmony with your natural design.
- A truly functional wardrobe requires ongoing maintenance, reflection, and mindset work as life continues to change.

Five

One Great Outfit

"Every once in a while a revolutionary product comes along that changes everything." - Steve Jobs

What if you didn't care what anyone else thought about what you were wearing?

I'd like to say that I never really cared much as to what other people thought about what I was wearing, but that would be a lie. A part of us always cares what other people think about us, because perceptions affect relationships, and none of us wants to be alone in life.

I can clearly recall wearing outfits in my teens out of pure love of style, and feeling a bit like I didn't fit in. In my junior year, I bought a black tracksuit with a rainbow stripe across the legs and chest and never had the right shoes for it. The best pair I had always made me feel kinda silly, but I wore them anyway because I loved the pants.

In ninth grade, I had an outfit of palazzo pants, a lace tee, and flowy vest because I saw a similar outfit on a senior and thought it was amazing. Nevermind that it looked too mature and my friends were all wearing original VSCO style (a mid-90s aesthetic recently revitalized) with oversized tees and boxer shorts. I even took my yearbook pictures in said outfit, immortalized forever in the way that only school pictures can be.

But in 2023, I experienced a style situation that forever changed my ability to care what others thought. For personal reasons, I began the practice of head covering—or wrapping my hair in a scarf. Women cover for a variety of reasons, from alopecia to religious convention, to simply enjoying the way it makes them feel. In my journey, I found a community filled with these different women, and a common struggle was managing other people's opinions of our choice.

I was incredibly nervous the first time I left the house with a scarf on my head. I wondered what other people would say and do, and if I would be treated differently. People close to me had strong reactions, often negative, that I had to field and face. Many women worried about actual violence and prejudice, but I was only concerned someone would make a rude comment to me.

My experience was actually the opposite of what we all feared: people held doors, strangers gave me compliments, and I had dozens of deeply meaningful conversations about my reasons. And even though my head covering practice has shifted, the lessons learned during that time of radical styling have stuck with me.

I learned that feeling completely confident in what we're wearing speaks volumes to everyone we meet. People react to us more authentically when we are being true to ourselves, and they don't really care much about what we're wearing.

That experience unlocked the true power of Youniform dressing. I realized it's not about the outfit at all...it's about freeing up mental space. When your wardrobe decisions are simplified and aligned, you stop worrying about how you look—because you *know* you look great, every day—and start focusing on living your life with passion and joy. You're no longer managing and obsessing over your appearance; instead, you are fully present in your life. That's the real power of an intentionally curated style.

When I first started trying to create capsule wardrobes, I tried to be like everyone else. I wasn't an expert, so even though I was trying to create something different, it was hard. Defaulting back to prescribed methods was easier. I branched out of just one dress into trying to build a skirt-based capsule wardrobe, with various types of skirts and shirts to mix and match.

But I hated it, and they just sat in my closet taking up space. I owned a lovely collection of clothing that I never wore. I always defaulted back to just one dress as the basis of my style. And every time, it made my life easier.

As we dive into the context of style uniforms—and the power of one great outfit—I'd like you to remember this idea of being so comfortable in our clothes that what other people think doesn't matter. Our easy clothing choice can become a vehicle for amazing conversations and interactions when our focus is on the people around us.

The Real Reason Successful People Repeat Outfits

On January 9, 2007, a man walked on stage to give a keynote presentation in San Francisco, California. Sources say he had practiced for days, like an actor preparing for a memorable role, down to the hand gestures (Gallo 2022). He promised a revolutionary product reveal, then teased the audience with three new tech devices.

As someone who meticulously planned the delivery, he left nothing to chance, including his clothing. But of all the things he designed, his outfit is likely the one that took the least amount of time.

Dressed in a simple, unadorned black mock-neck tee, medium-wash jeans, and black sneakers, Steve Jobs took the stage and announced the development of one of the greatest technological advancements of our generation: the iPhone.

Just as his invention became the foundational backbone of modern smartphones, so too has his iconic outfit become the base for our understanding of a style Youniform. His identifiable black turtleneck, jeans, and sneakers are found in photos dating back to 1998. From that time until his death, Apple released the iPod (2001), MacBook (2006), Apple TV & iPhone (2007), and the iPad (2010), along with numerous other tech hardware developments, and he wore the same thing each time. You can easily say that his simple style choice had an inverse relationship with his creative output: the less he thought about what to wear, the more space he had to think about changing the world.

After studying dozens of high-impact women—leaders, visionaries, and creators intent on leaving their mark—I've found the same pattern holds true. The simpler their daily style decisions, the more energy they have to focus on the work that matters.

Streamlining what you wear isn't about minimalism; it's about mastery. It's a quiet act of alignment of your wardrobe that allows you to invest your mental resources in purpose rather than presentation.

But what exactly is a style Youniform?

In its most basic definition, it's literally wearing the exact same thing every day, purchased in duplicate. Steve Jobs likely had multiple black tops and pairs of jeans. Mark Zuckerberg has commented on his closet filled with the same gray tee and jeans. My grandfather had a closet filled with the same seven blue button-downs and seven pairs of jeans.

The. Exact. Same. Thing. On. Repeat.

You could take this route. You could stop reading right now and commit to wearing the same thing every single day. Maybe it's jeans and a tee like these tech CEOs. Maybe it's the same navy dress. Or perhaps gray slacks and a light blue button-up work perfectly for you.

I have personally used this route once for a "micro" Youniform: In 2009 I was incredibly busy and adopted the black tee and jeans for my weekend Youniform. Another time, I wore the same black dress for 100 days as a personal style challenge.

But in my day-to-day life, I find this to be a bit too constricting. So instead, I'm going to be sharing how to make this more custom for the rest of this chapter.

For now, ask yourself what your core style Youniform would be. If you were forced to wear the exact same thing every day, *a la* Steve Jobs, what would be your default Youniform? I want you to get a picture in your head, because it probably says a lot about your base style preferences.

You Need More Than a Black Tee and Jeans

I love the color black. I consider it an easy default and love that it forms a blank canvas for other bold colors. As a winter, I'm fortunate that it also looks good on me, but after wearing it for 100 days straight, I'll admit to being burnt out. After that experiment, I wore navy for a good six months instead, because the black felt too austere.

For most of us, the idea of the exact same thing every day feels too constricting, whether it's black or gray or even yellow. Men seem not to have this aversion, as many stories of personal Youniform dressing involve men like Jobs or Zuckerberg (or my husband, who is happy with one sage green tee and the same jeans).

A Youniform doesn't limit your expression; it refines it.

Women often experience clothing differently than men. Men don't dress for each other, but women do—and we all know it. There's an unspoken rule that women are evaluated more closely, more often, and usually by other women. And as we get older, that pressure shifts. Society makes women feel invisible with age, and many of us instinctively use clothing to stay seen. Dressing well becomes a form of self-preservation, a quiet way of saying, *I'm still here.*

And regardless of what other people might think, we also want to enjoy the experience of wearing our clothes. At the time I'm writing this, "dopamine dressing" has become a hot keyword, and refers to choosing clothes that make us feel good or bring us joy—releasing the feel-good hormone dopamine.

But this desire for variety and beauty is exactly why I developed a different approach—one that simplifies the decision making while still allowing you to choose clothes that bring you joy and happiness.

A Youniform doesn't limit your expression; it refines it.

It gives you the clarity of a logical system and the freedom to express your most authentic self through style.

The question then became: what if we could capture all the benefits of Youniform dressing while still expressing our creativity and individuality? That question led me to develop the Youniform Framework—my signature process for taking the genius of a style Youniform and multiplying it through color and lifestyle application.

Over five years of working with hundreds of women with different styles, I tested and refined this approach through real-world application. What started as a personal experiment became a proven system that my clients now use to create 64+ outfit combinations from just twelve carefully chosen pieces.

The Youniform Framework is a multifaceted approach that uses the first three style stages of color, style, and fit, to design a complete wardrobe for every single part of life. We use color to create cohesion and repetition in our personal uniforms. Your unique style personality and fit requirements are used to build outfits that look stunning without obsessing over how to pair this top with that skirt. And your "right now" lifestyle needs dictate how many and what types of uniforms you create to get you through the week.

Because your life needs more than one black tee and pair of jeans every day. Like Marsha, who needed comfy clothes for retirement and activewear for traveling with her grandkids. Or Miranda, who needed two separate church outfits to express her style after a week of required work uniforms.

And then there's Dawn, a long-time client who wore a tee and jeans outfit for years, naturally gravitating to Youniform dressing. As much as we want to dress for joy and growth, life isn't always beautiful, and sometimes it throws a lot at us at once. Several months ago Dawn suddenly lost her husband in a car accident. The shock was overwhelming and the grief was immediate.

In the weeks following, she was bombarded with the legal and logistical realities of her new life, all while trying to steady herself emotionally. With her permission, I share her story: she told me how being able to grab multiple Youniform types (pants, dresses, and pajamas) without thinking made space for her to handle the enormity of bringing closure to her husband's affairs. Instead of having to make involved clothing choices each day (or stay messy in pajamas), she was free to focus on the daunting decisions that came up. We can always hope for beauty, but even in the darkest moments, the clothes we wear can make life easier or harder.

Each of us has a unique schedule that requires different clothes. What works for someone else won't work for you, which is why those prescribed capsule wardrobes and essentials lists fail you. Think about the implications of what's in your closet. If you don't need a blazer, is there any reason to have even one in your closet? How often do *you* wear a little black dress? Instead of buying one-offs for special events, we could always borrow them or find what we need.

The Youniform Framework teaches you to curate your closet based on You Essentials—only the clothing pieces needed to live your life fully. You plan each outfit carefully and repeat them using a simple method, which ensures beautiful variety (so don't worry; no one will ever think you wear the same thing every day!).

Mornings are easy because you assess your daily activities and pick the corresponding outfit for maximum impact. Your biggest decision becomes what color you're in the mood to wear. The daily requirement to get dressed is no longer stressful, and you get to save your decision-making power for more important things.

Before we move on, I'd like you to think about a number.

If you consider just a single style Youniform for one aspect of your life, how many items do you think you would need to make it work? Would it be seven? Five? Ten? Now think about that in relation to the other areas of your life where you need a Youniform and reconsider that number. Next, I'll show you a simple formula for answering that question.

How to Create Variety in a Style Youniform

Since we've established that you don't want to own seven black tees and jeans because you want more variety, it's time to get into exactly what that looks like in practice.

I know this might feel overwhelming—especially after realizing how much mental energy you've been wasting on outfit decisions—but I promise this next method will feel like a relief. We will do this using a method I like to call the 4-Piece Wardrobe. Don't let the name fool you, it's not about owning four items of clothing. Four specific pieces will become the structure for building an outfit module that gives you sixty-four different combinations, ensuring that you could go two months in a single style uniform without repeating.

I developed this method when I finally stopped forcing variety and finally committed to a dress-only wardrobe. I had already learned how to make many wardrobe choices with a few colors, so I used that idea here

I decided on two neutral and two color dresses per season (sixteen dresses total). I used the same format with completer pieces to expand the structure and variety. Around the same time, I noticed a pattern with my Youniform clients: they naturally gravitated toward three or four favorite color combinations, and everything else in their closet was just noise. Their preferences validated what I had discovered. To this day, I still love showing women how one simple Youniform built on the 4-Piece Wardrobe method can create sixty-four unique outfit variations.

The 4-Piece Wardrobe is a way of building out each personal Youniform by collecting four of each outfit component: 4 tops, 4 bottoms, and 4 completer pieces. There are a few more specifics that make this work easily. For the sake of teaching, it's easiest to describe this process using concrete ideas. Follow along with me as I build out an easy jeans and tee Youniform as an example.

We always start with bottoms, because they are the most difficult item to get "right."

After working with hundreds of clients, I've seen that finding the right fit in jeans or skirts takes the most time. Because sizing and fit are inconsistent for women, they create frustration and wasted energy. But the flow of the entire outfit depends on the foundation, so we front-load the styling effort by starting with the biggest challenge. In this case we are choosing jeans, but we must be specific in our styling choices to make this work. Let's go ahead and name our client Caitlin so we can keep track.

Caitlin likes her jeans to be middle-of-the-road in style, so, straight cut and mid-rise is her preference. The 4-Piece Wardrobe says that we begin by collecting four of this same style pant. If you can shop at the same retailer, this is always best, as their clothing will be the most similar and make getting dressed a breeze. But if not, getting specific about the style details is the next best thing.

The 4-Piece Wardrobe uses a specific color framework to make this process varied and highly individual. At its core, the focus is on two neutrals and two colors, but we can take some liberty with this as we move along. Back to Caitlin's jeans: we're going to follow this framework exactly, but later I'll show you how to tweak it a bit for your own taste.

Caitlin is a Soft Autumn, so our color selections will be warm-neutral, medium to dark value, and muted or soft. Four pairs of straight-leg jeans could be a medium-wash denim (neutral 1), a soft cream/ivory (neutral 2), a warm olive (color 1), and a rich burgundy (color 2).

***Pro tip*: once you find a retailer whose clothes consistently fit you well, stick with them. Fit consistency saves hours of frustration and gives you confidence that anything you order will work with the rest of your wardrobe. Building a relationship with a trusted brand allows you to spend less time guessing and more time enjoying how your clothes make you feel.**

With the bottoms portion of the Youniform completed, it's time to move our attention to the tops. Caitlin prefers V-neck tops to give breathing room for her shoulders and has found one retailer that she loves, so all of her purchases will be at one place for these. This is the part where having a good grasp of color is critical to making sure all four tops will work with all four bottoms. Choosing hot pink here would be a color-matching disaster. But Caitlin is solid in her color choices, so her four tops are chocolate brown (neutral 1), soft beige (neutral 2), muted gold (color 1), and deep forest green (color 2).

Here, we could have used the same colors for the pants, but I want to demonstrate how color theory allows for easy matching even with many different colors. We could stop here and Caitlin would be able to make sixteen outfits from her eight items of clothing:

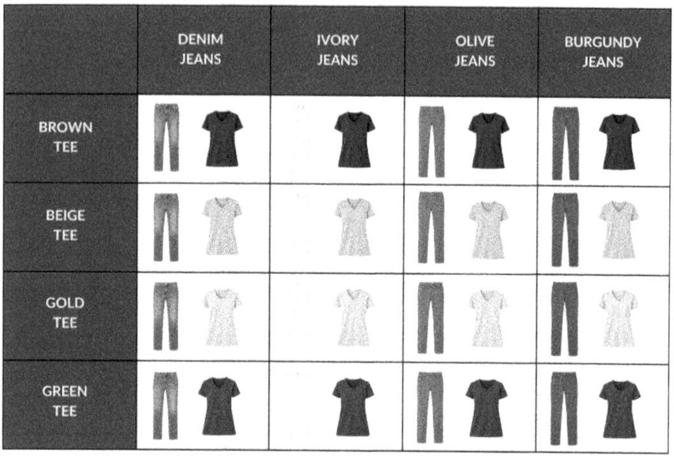

Table 5.1 Graphical depiction of how eight items of clothing combine into sixteen outfits in a Youniform (for full color images visit youniformbook.com)

This is before we add completer pieces to finish the look, which is going to take us up to sixty-four outfits. Because we have all solids, we're going to make the first adaptation to the 4-Piece Wardrobe by substituting one of the color selections with a print.

Caitlin is using this personal Youniform for a casual everyday weekend look and prefers a long open cardigan to keep it comfortable. We want to mimic some of the other colors in her existing pieces to avoid her looking like a rainbow and to help the eye settle, so her cardigan colors will be Ivory (neutral 1), tan (neutral 2), olive (color 1), and a botanical print cardigan featuring shades of peach, rose, and burgundy (color 2).

At this point, Caitlin's casual jeans Youniform is complete, with four pairs of straight-leg jeans, four V-neck tees, and four open cardigans, all selected using a framework of two neutral color selections and two color selections. She can mix and match all the pieces to give the same Youniform, but now she has variety and fun that speaks to her own sense of style. She still benefits from easy outfit selection when she gets dressed, even if it's not all the same black tee like Steve Jobs.

Adding her four completer pieces to her eight style-base items allows her to create a total of sixty-four outfit combinations. Only a small portion of people would ever catch on that she's essentially wearing the same thing every day, because she has used color and a bit of a print to add depth and nuance to her style Youniform.

One of my clients recently shared how this system completely changed her Sundays. She told me she used to obsess over what to wear to church each week, trying on multiple outfits and feeling flustered before leaving the house. Now, she gets dressed peacefully every Sunday morning and receives compliments almost every week on her beautiful print tops, even from the teens in the nursery. Her style didn't change; she just refined it to a place of confidence and now gets to show up more focused on others.

I want to share a few more examples, taking greater latitude with the 4-Piece Wardrobe and applying it to a more formal setting.

For the first, I'll use myself as an example. I wear dresses 99% of the time, and I really love a good print dress. Most of my dresses follow a fit and flare style, keeping the silhouette the same. You might think that I can't use this framework with a print, but it's easy to apply it with a bit of thought on how prints work.

Since prints are essentially a variety of color choices, I can use this color framework in the following way: black and white check print (neutral 1), gray and white damask print (neutral 2), green and white stripe print (color 1), and floral print with teal base and multicolored flowers (color 2). We are keeping the same framework, but adapting it to focus on the base color of each style and the amount of color in the actual print.

Moving on, I prefer a wrap-style cardigan, and since all the dresses are print, I will stick to solid colors here: black (neutral 1), midnight navy (neutral 2), deep plum (color 1), Aegean teal (color 2). All my colors share the same attributes: cool-neutral, medium to deep value, slightly bright so I can easily pair the green or teal print with plum and teal, and yes, I do wear black and navy together!

You may have noticed that I cannot create sixty-four combinations, since I am working with a two-piece style Youniform. This is a great time to talk about making it work for your needs.

The 4-Piece Wardrobe is a guideline, and there are no style police telling you that you can't add more than this. It's about keeping balance in your color choices to keep the Youniform easily mixable. If you need six of each item, choose three neutrals, and three colors. If, like me, the dress Youniform is your workhorse, maybe having 12 dresses makes more sense, and half of them are neutral-based while the other half are color-based. You can still stick to four completer pieces or add a few more if needed (I have six and it's perfect).

But if you are creating multiple style Youniforms, starting with your most used and sticking to the 4-Piece Wardrobe is going to give you loads of mileage in your closet.

I'll share one more example for a more formal office setting. Suppose Amanda is a partner working in a legal office that still prefers a business professional wardrobe. She finds two-piece pantsuits easy to buy and use in her closet, so we use that as the framework to begin.

Amanda is a Soft Summer and black makes her look washed out, but she needs the formality of acceptable neutrals. For her suits, we will adapt to her needs and stick with neutrals in this way: solid navy suit (neutral 1), solid gray suit (neutral 2), subtle gray herringbone suit (neutral print 1), navy pinstripe suit (neutral print 2). We have added variety here by adding very subtle, classic prints that are acceptable in a formal office setting.

We will add more variety to her tops by choosing suitable neutrals and colors . To keep it streamlined and simple, she wears simple silk short-sleeve tops under her suits. To keep with her color scheme, we choose a light and dark neutral of ivory and navy, along with a cornflower blue (color 1) and a blush pink (color 2).

With a five day workweek, Amanda might add one more suit to cover the entire week, and another color top or two for variety. Or perhaps her firm does business casual Friday, and she can mix in a fun blazer with any of her suiting pants, or mix it up with a dress.

The 4-Piece Wardrobe creates the framework for adding variety to any style Youniform you create. It allows you to create a modular system of wearing the same thing on repeat, maximizing the benefit of repeatable outfits while making sure that your unique style and preference speaks.

Take a quick survey of what you're wearing right now and ask yourself if it could be a style Youniform. Could you add pieces following the two neutral and two color rule to create a repeatable set of outfits that you love wearing?

One Youniform = 384 Days of Style

When we were creating Amanda's formal business outfit, you may have noticed I slipped in a few extras there at the end. The final exploration of the Youniform Framework speaks to how to add some variety to the core of your style Youniform. This goes beyond adding more tops or bottoms or even the same style of completer pieces into things like one-off items: shoes, jewelry, and other accessories. If she loves scarves, she might've added some high-end prints or chosen some colorful shoes for a pop of fun.

I'm a cardigan girl, through and through. I like them soft and flowy and cozy enough that if I decide to take a mid-afternoon nap, I can lie down in them and sleep. But sometimes it's nice to have something a little different. Therefore, I have a few different items, such as a denim jacket or leather jacket, that I can substitute when needed.

Switching out a completer piece is the first way that we can add variety to our basic setup of tops and bottoms to get more mileage out of the outfit. In the first example above, Caitlin could decide to switch up her options by adding a flowy vest or kimono in a print, and a corduroy shacket in ivory plaid to get a few more options. She somewhat mimics the shape of her cardigan to make sure that the silhouette and lines of her Youniform stay the same.

But this also brings up a major question: what about when the weather changes? Caitlin wanted to keep it simple with jeans and a V-neck top. The cardigans give her coverage for many of the fluctuations of spring and fall, but what about summer and winter? Assuming that her top is a short sleeve, she could swap out her jeans for shorts in a similar rise and preferred inseam, choosing some lighter colors like light denim, beige, peach, and banana. She is able to keep all her tops consistent with these and might get more use out of the light completer mentioned above, or even adding more.

When winter comes, she can swap out the short-sleeve tees for long-sleeve versions, or even similar-style sweaters in darker colors like espresso, cognac, forest green, and burgundy. She could add the shacket we added afterwards or pull in a vest since her arms are now covered and warm. Her jeans will continue to work with these updates to the tops.

When switching between cool and warm calendar seasons, it's important to mimic the shapes and details of the original Youniform. In doing so, we explode our options for mixing and matching as we move from a basic design of four tops and bottoms to eight tops and bottoms that cover temperature fluctuations. Now our outfit count is at sixty-four with no completers and adding two more of those for six total means that we now have 384 outfit ideas out of a very basic set of clothing.

That's enough to mix and match twenty-two items of clothing for a full year without repeating a single combo—suddenly the idea of one great outfit makes sense in a whole new way! But we're not even done adding the extras.

Beyond the clothing we wear on our actual bodies, the small additions of shoes, jewelry, and other accessories add variety to our outfits. If we consider just two seasons to keep it simple (spring/summer and fall/winter, aka warm and cool), we can continue to add dimension to one great outfit by choosing eight pairs of shoes for the entire year.

Choose a mix of shoes for different occasions, from casual to sporty to dressy to active, to get a large range out of one basic Youniform. In Caitlin's case, for cool weather she might choose two pairs of boots, loafers, and a pair of heeled booties. For warm weather perhaps two pairs of sandals, flats, and fashion sneakers. As she chooses these in colors that complement her Soft Autumn wardrobe, she gets more interest with her outfits and can wear them in more situations.

An outfit is never complete without some jewelry to make it look intentional, and well-styled. Jewelry selections are year-round items, but having a basic Youniform for shiny baubles is helpful too. To cover many uses, she could have at minimum two pairs each of earrings, necklaces, and bracelets to wear with her simple jeans Youniform. As a lover of earrings, I personally have the exact same style in six different colors to go with all my outfits. Jewelry speaks volumes, so don't forget this step in executing your one great outfit.

There are other accessories that can be planned and added to finalize a well-rounded uniform module. Fabric goods like scarves, leather goods like belts, the purse that we choose to carry, and even small items like hair accessories or keychains can add more dimension to our overall presentation of style. Each area can be mindfully curated using the same 4-Piece Wardrobe framework as a baseline for understanding how to add using color in a controlled and cohesive way.

Once we make these additions, the ability to maximize one simple Youniform becomes exponential. You may never have considered how one simple outfit could become the backbone of an entire year-round wardrobe, but it's possible, and you don't have to have all black to make it functional.

As we close this chapter, I'd like to invite you to explore the potential outcome of this concept in comparison with what you're wearing right now. Earlier I asked you to consider whether it could be your personal Youniform if you multiplied it. Now I want you to think about how you could modify it throughout the year, what kind of alternate completer pieces would you want, what types of shoes would you mix and match, what is your favorite jewelry to wear, and how might a great purse in your signature color make it all pop?

As you envision your own 4-Piece Wardrobe, notice how different this feels from standing in your closet feeling overwhelmed. This is what it feels like when your wardrobe finally serves your vision instead of stealing your energy. You're no longer dressing for convenience or expectation, but with clarity and intention. You're no longer thinking of yourself as someone who struggles with clothes, but as someone who has found the secret to dressing well with a purpose, and without effort.

If you're ready to put this into practice, grab your free copy of the Youniform Planner at **youniformbook.com**. Inside you'll find a spreadsheet that helps you design your first 4-Piece Wardrobe and start curating your own lifestyle uniforms. This simple step will help you turn today's ideas into tomorrow's clarity. As you work through it, remember that every choice you make now is paving the way for peaceful mornings, effortless style, and exponential impact.

And as you'll see in the next chapter, there's one more piece to complete the picture, your unique lifestyle and rhythm. It's the part of the process that ensures that your Youniforms fit every role, responsibility, and rhythm of your real life.

Chapter Five Highlights

- True style confidence comes from wearing clothes that feel fully aligned with who you are, not from managing other people's opinions.
- Repeating a great outfit is not laziness or minimalism, but a strategic way to reduce decision fatigue and protect mental energy.
- A style Youniform works because it shifts attention away from appearance and toward purpose, presence, and meaningful work.
- The 4-Piece Wardrobe creates a repeatable outfit structure by using four coordinated pieces to generate dozens of combinations.
- The Youniform Framework preserves creativity and joy while eliminating daily outfit stress.
- One well-designed Youniform can support an entire year of life by adapting to seasons, settings, and emotional bandwidth.

Six

7 Outfits for Life

"All life is an experiment. The more experiments you make, the better." - Ralph Waldo Emerson

I love to shop. But even more than the experience of shopping, I love to *collect.*

In my mind, there was an ideal wardrobe setup, and I was determined to find it. After completing my 100-day dress challenge, I started transitioning my entire wardrobe to merino wool, but things spiraled out of hand. This path of sustainability offered so many new brands I had never met, and just like Pokemon, I had to catch them all.

I don't want to think about how much money I spent in the year following the challenge...the one that was supposed to show me how much better off I was with less. The irony is that I just traded the addiction of fast fashion for that of slow fashion. But an addiction is still an addiction.

My closet was fabulous and sustainable, but I couldn't wear it all. It had become a collection to display that made me happy just for owning it. But our clothes should be functional, and things that we're wearing to live our lives to the fullest. Even though my closet wasn't bloated by average standards, it had become excessive for me.

As I wrestled with the dawning reality of what I was doing, I considered the option of a no-buy year. A dear friend was experiencing the same recognition, and we tossed about the idea as an option to fix our obsession with shopping. I read a book around this time from a woman who completed a no-buy clothing year, and her experience impressed me.

I decided to try this experiment, which I knew would be difficult, starting the day after my birthday. Admittedly, I just wanted one last chance to shop with abandon. I designated it a "low-buy" instead of no-buy and gave myself parameters and lists and allowable purchases throughout the year. It was difficult, but after the first month I stopped obsessing about shopping and stalking my favorite retailers. My sense of personal style got even clearer based on using what I had and noticing what I ignored.

About six months in, life threw a wrench in my plans with a pregnancy. I had gotten rid of 99% of my maternity clothes because they were separates and also because I *thought* we were done (lesson learned). So, I knew I would have to bend the rules I had created for function before my year was over. But I had already changed so much that I could handle the whole pregnancy with no need for a new maternity wardrobe.

Forcing myself to quit shopping constantly removed the dopamine hit I was getting from collecting clothes. It allowed me to appreciate what I had and get rid of what I wasn't using. Instead of fixing my style frustrations with something new, I had to get creative with what was in my closet, which helped me refine what

I loved even more. During this forced experiment, the concept of my four-piece wardrobe solidified. I noticed that even though I owned seven versions of certain items, the same three or four favorites kept showing up in the laundry basket week after week. That realization became a turning point: *extra isn't better; it's just excess.*

You may not realize the powerful hold that the fashion industry has over all of us. Their wealth is staggering, and their constant message to *buy buy buy* to keep up is overwhelming. Fashion houses release collections at a blistering pace, and yesterday's trends are already outdated. Frequent shopping for clothes dulls your senses to what you actually want and need.

Remember from Chapter One that the average woman wears only about 10% of her wardrobe, yet continues purchasing new items every other week. For busy women juggling careers, homes, and purpose-driven goals, this endless shopping cycle isn't harmless fun. It drains both finances and mental clarity, stealing the time and focus that you could invest in what truly matters.

Even a capsule wardrobe or a minimalist wardrobe can become a trap if we fall into the habit of constantly collecting and seeking perfection. In the previous chapters, you identified a primary Youniform and saw how one great outfit can become the blueprint for your style. In this chapter, we are going to zoom out and turn that single outfit into an entire wardrobe system that supports your real life from every angle.

Most women do not live in only one context. Work, home, family, church, and social events all intermingle with rest. That means most women need more than one Youniform. Here, you will learn how to use your lifestyle audit to decide which parts of your week actually deserve their own Youniform so you can build a small set of reliable "go-to" looks instead of trying to be prepared for every possible scenario.

There will be no blazers or cocktail dresses "just in case," and if you hate button-down shirts, you won't own one. I want you to think logically about the life you're living right now (not yesterday or tomorrow), and decide accordingly. Just like when I had to make a few tweaks for pregnancy, you'll learn how to craft and design a closet for your life today.

What No One Tells You About Capsule Wardrobes

I fell in love with capsule wardrobes in 2015. This was the first time I had heard this term. I was pregnant (it's a theme, okay?), and it seemed amazing. Project 333 was my introduction, and with a maternity wardrobe it's easy to designate thirty-three items and move on with life. Afterwards, I found working with a capsule wardrobe so hard because I had too many options.

When I created the Youniform Framework, it stemmed from my desire for a customized capsule wardrobe, with parameters and a process for curating. I use it as a specialized type of capsule wardrobe, but some of my clients use it from a more maximalist perspective. The beauty of this system is that you can use it for minimalism, maximalism, or anything in between. It gives you control and guidance over the clothes you need, and how to build a functional closet with clear steps and stages.

These two concepts—capsule and module—present similarities and differences. If you're familiar with capsule wardrobes, you'll be able to see how Youniforms evolved through the process. And if you've never heard of them, this will be my version of your education into capsules.

A capsule wardrobe is a thoughtfully curated collection of clothing that emphasizes quality over quantity, aimed at simplifying life and streamlining daily routines. While it can be minimalistic, the focus is more on having a smaller, more manageable set of clothing items. These should be clothes that you love and that reflect your personal style and lifestyle needs. It's a strategic way of dressing that helps you make the most out of every item in your closet, ensuring each piece has a purpose and a place in your everyday life.

So far, the Youniform Framework meets all the requirements here, which is why it's a form of a capsule wardrobe—but better! Both a traditional capsule wardrobe and a Youniform:

- Aim to simplify your wardrobe and daily outfit choices
- Focus on limiting the range of items for less clutter and easier decisions
- Center on the use of mix-and-match pieces for versatile outfit creation
- Encourage sustainability and contentment with fewer, higher-quality items

One of the biggest struggles I had trying to implement Project 333 was the lack of guidance. Choose thirty-three items and wear them for three months...ok, cool. But what thirty-three items? How many pairs of shoes should I have? What about pants or tops, and what if I have thirty-four items?! Does that mean I'm a capsule wardrobe failure? You can find all these questions on forums discussed tirelessly by those who are trying to follow the process.

Some people embrace vague concepts, but many of us need a plan that makes sense. This is where the Youniform Framework differs from a capsule wardrobe.

The Youniform Framework helps you build what we'll call a modular wardrobe, so you can stop questioning your choices and focusing on arbitrary numbers. We suggest you start with something like the 4-Piece Wardrobe, but that is your basic framework, and you should adapt it if necessary.

Another key Youniform difference is the focus on detailed repetition of styles and silhouettes. I love scrolling through Pinterest® and looking at those beautiful curated capsule wardrobe idea pins. They are visually striking, but filled with neutrals that make little sense for every skin tone, and a confusing variety of clothing types to put together. Trying to pair different cuts of shirts with the same type of pants is a recipe for morning frustration.

Our personal body lines are unique and favor certain silhouettes to truly shine, but imposing different outfit silhouettes on it makes us feel frumpy and dowdy. The Youniform Framework focuses on finding your style and making your closet consistent, rather than offering a wide range of options. The focus is on creating go-to outfits or personal uniforms instead of the mix-and-match outfit system of a traditional capsule wardrobe.

Finally, The Youniform Framework is a complete education system, not just a theoretical concept. I have read many style books with transformational information, but the implementation lacked clarity. When I went looking for a deeper application, there existed only public chat rooms debating the topic. The book was the end of the knowledge.

I built the Youniform Framework in the trenches (alongside my wonderful clients), and it goes through updates as needed. With each version comes new training and tools to make the process easy to apply. That's why I created an entire suite of products around the Youniform Framework. From do-it-yourself spreadsheets to personalized guidance in our group style coaching program, we want everyone to have access to apply this wisdom.

Visit younifórmbook.com to get all the free resources we've included with your book, including the Youniform Planner, plus other tools to help you get started implementing what you've learned.

Whether you choose the simplicity of one great outfit like Steve Jobs (but more fun), or you need seven great outfits because your life is crazy busy, the Youniform Framework will give you support and guidance as you curate a closet that lets you live your life fully and with purpose.

The Style System Hidden in Your Routine

2009 will go down in my memory as one of the busiest times of my life (pre-kids at least). After finishing my bachelor's degree, I took a job in hospital administration and worked a nine-to-five. I lived in a micro-town, and my commute was forty-five minutes each way back when gas spiked over $4/gallon in Texas. I was also working on my MBA in the evenings a few nights a week, bored through accounting and overwhelmed in quantitative analysis.

Then, I fell in love with scuba diving. I had read about it in books for over a decade, and it always seemed like an amazing experience. The first time I tried it, I was hooked. Even though I lived in a landlocked town, I fed my obsession with continued diving education and finally became a divemaster. (I eventually ended up burning down that crazy-busy life and moving to Florida to become a dive bum, but that's a story for another day.)

One requirement of training was a timed swim, so my day began by getting up around 4:45 am, driving forty-five minutes to the gym, swimming a mile, showering and getting dressed for work, then fueling up on coffee before either an evening business class or dive class. Weekends were just for diving, waking up early, packing bags and coolers, driving 2-3 hours to a tiny murky lake, and spending all day in the water. There was little downtime, but I was blissfully exhausted at the end of each day.

Looking back, this was the first time that I heavily implemented style Youniforms in my life for simplicity. I was doing the same things all the time, and having repeatable outfits for each event saved me time during a phase when I had very little to spare. I was burning the candle at both ends so hard I didn't realize at the time how much energy I was saving. As a woman trying to "live the dream"—career, education, fitness, and passions—the last thing I needed was to waste precious brain power on what to wear. But most women I know are still fighting this battle every day.

This principle established the Youniform Framework as outfit modules. A module is defined as a set of parts that when combined, make a whole. Each 4-Piece Wardrobe we design becomes the basis for a single outfit module. We can analyze the activities of our current life to discover how many of these modules we need to get dressed easily for any situation. And when we apply the principles of color and silhouette, we can ensure that the individual pieces from each module can play with other module pieces.

During my insane grad school diving days, I had about four Youniform modules, with some being large and others minimalist leaning:

- I had a swim Youniform, consisting of a Speedo suit, Under Armour running shorts, and logo tees from a local athletic shop. I usually paired these with flip flops and I wore it to the pool, changed into a rash guard when diving to stay covered, and added jeans afterward. This one stayed fairly true to the 4-Piece Wardrobe in quantity.

- My work Youniform was a bit more varied. I wore wide-leg slacks in black and charcoal and had an assortment of lightweight knit tops. A few funky and mod non-blazer jackets added a professional edge, and I rotated through my extensive collection of heels.

- On the weekends when I wasn't diving, I was tired, so I defaulted to Steve Jobs with jeans and a quality black tee. I recall having three black tees and just two pairs of designer jeans.

- Finally, I had a micro Youniform for those occasions when my friends and I went out for dinner or drinks. Either a dress or a fancy top with those jeans I mentioned. I definitely had fewer than four in quantity for this module.

My schedule was the same from week to week. I was in the groove of living my life, doing what was meaningful to me and my closet was a workhorse in getting me there. I have come to realize that our lives are repetitive in nature; we do the same things all the time for long seasons. Eventually, we shift and have a new set of requirements for which we need Youniforms.

I am going to help you explore the various areas of your life so you can clearly identify where you need to create repeatable style uniforms. Each one of these will become its own outfit module, designed to function optimally for a set of circumstances. Right now as you're reading this book, take a look at what you're wearing. Analyze the pieces of your outfit and consider all the areas where it would be perfect. Maybe it's loungewear just for being at home. Maybe you're at a coffee shop, and it's a casual everyday look. Or maybe you're on your lunch break and you're wearing your work Youniform. Your life already has a schedule and a rhythm, and we're going to go over it and find the places where a Youniform fits.

Create the Perfect Youniform for Every Moment

Perhaps you're so busy running around like a chicken with its head cut off like I was, that you've never thought about your life by grouping activities. But that is exactly the first step in figuring out exactly what your closet needs to help you live a life of purpose.

So far, we've looked at utilizing one great outfit as a primary style Youniform. I want to reiterate that *this can be enough*. It worked for Steve Jobs, and it could work for you too if you wanted it to. If you don't have a wide variety of social gatherings or complex wardrobe requirements, a well-designed single style Youniform with a few more than four pieces will take you through most things. But what about those who have many wardrobe needs?

This is where the Youniform Framework shines, because each person can customize the process for their unique life and needs. All of our important and mundane moments get the pleasure of having the perfect outfit to match. Most women find that 3-5 Youniforms is a good number to have. The next step is figuring out where there is overlap in our lives and what those outfits will be.

The best way to uncover this information is through a Lifestyle Audit. This is a process of combing through your activities over a given time period and writing it all down. This doesn't take long and should provide clarity about the things you're currently involved in doing. It's worth noting that this process is designed to show you what you need clothes for right now.

Dressing a past self or a non-existent fantasy version of yourself has no room in this process. Many women I meet are using their closets as storage space for clothes they haven't worn in a decade "just in case". I often meet other clients who impulse buy items for unknown reasons, usually because it seems more interesting than their current life. I want to remind you that the life you have today is the life you're supposed to have. Whether it's insanely busy or seems boring and uneventful, it's the place where you belong today. And you deserve to look and feel your best.

I had one client, Alice, who had stunning clothes and loved to shop for beautiful treasures—but many of them simply weren't practical for caring for her adult son with special needs. She kept defaulting to casual, cozy clothes and felt like something was wrong with her because of it. One day I finally gave her permission to dress for the life she was living, and together we built an entire Youniform for her life that was both flattering and functional. Every day after that Alice felt less pressured to wear everything and more at ease to be herself living her amazing life.

Let's go back to Amanda, our attorney, to illustrate how a Lifestyle Audit works in real time. Her business professional attire through the week has already been established, which takes up a good portion of her time every week. Upon examination of her monthly schedule, she also has these things scheduled: personal training each week before work, a fundraising gala, tickets to the theater, brunch with her sorority sisters, a volunteer day at her local women's shelter, a family dinner for her dad's birthday, and one guest speaking event for a professional organization for female attorneys.

By looking at her various activities, we can see some similarities and group them into those that might require a similar personal Youniform. The gala and the theater both require a level of formality, so formal wear is one of her Youniforms. The fitness needs will require a specific Youniform, and the speaking event can use her business Youniform with potential tweaks as mentioned before. Her social needs, like brunch and family dinner, could use the same Youniform, and the volunteer day might illustrate a need for something more low-key.

With her work Youniform complete, we can now identify the additional Youniforms Amanda needs to support the rest of her weekly rhythm. Quickly we can ideate the options for each of these areas:

- **Formal Youniform** - with varying degrees of formality, Amanda keeps cocktail dresses in charcoal and dusty mauve. For black-tie events like the gala, she chooses to rent designer gowns as needed. Her formal wear Youniform contains a couple of pairs of heels, formal clutch, decorative jewelry, and a few wrap and coat options for warmth.

- **Fitness Youniform** - Amanda is focused on weightlifting for bone health, so she needs fitness clothing that is fitted to allow for movement and form checks from her trainer. She has a favorite athletic wear retailer, so she purchases workout leggings in gray and navy, and tanks in neutrals and colors. She has a couple of lightweight zip hoodies to wear when transitioning, plus two pairs of zero-drop sneakers.

- **Social Youniform** - since she wears pants to work, she likes to be more feminine for her friends and family get-togethers. For this, she chooses sheath dresses and has a mix of colors and prints to keep it light and fun. Since these are more casual, she adds flat footwear to the mix, like sandals for warm weather and loafers for a closed-toe option. She also includes some colorful fashion jewelry and uses high-quality cardigans if layering is needed.

- **Low-Key Youniform** - for her volunteer activities, simple weekend events, and relaxing around the house, she sticks with classic jeans and a well-fitting tee. She buys the exact same pair of jeans in the same wash in duplicate and chooses an assortment of tees based on the 4-Piece Wardrobe. A pair of fashion sneakers completes the outfit, and she can use layers and jewelry from other areas to change the vibe.

With this plan complete, Amanda is dressed for anything life throws at her. She no longer worries about what to wear, because she knows exactly what her life needs and what clothing works for every event. As she gets dressed each day, she reviews the schedule in her head, and grabs the most appropriate clothing, putting together outfits that are already planned and work together based on cohesive color choices. She gets to focus on purpose and impact, instead of spending her mental energy on the clothes she is wearing.

A Lifestyle Audit is a simple exercise that you can use to get clarity on your own style needs right now. Take a few minutes and review the next month and what you have planned. Consider the one-off events but also carefully think through an average "boring" day, from what you do in the morning to how you spend your evening downtime. All of your activities deserve the perfect style solution.

Once you have noted all the activities, look for areas of overlap where you could use the same outfit configuration and group your needs. It's likely you will end up with 3-5 different personal Youniforms for your current life.

Then celebrate! Your wardrobe needs should seem much more clear at this very moment. You've done some great work so far, and you should be able to envision how adopting Youniforms across your life could simplify getting dressed, while also making you feel great, and making sure that your energy and focus is on the things that matter, versus what you're wearing.

The Only Seven Outfits You'll Ever Need

For years I taught the Lifestyle Audit as the path to determining exactly what you need. But I had many clients get stuck here, unable to clearly communicate what they needed for their life. I see this a lot, especially in women who deal with perfectionism. They cannot take a step back, view the process from a 30,000ft perspective, and make decisive decisions about each area.

I'll admit that I love creating frameworks that address these kinds of struggles with a concrete system. After analyzing the common lifestyle needs of my clients over five years, the Lifestyle Audit evolved into a clear framework for creating easy to categorize outfits. One day, after answering the same questions about cardigans for what felt like the millionth time, it finally clicked: my clients needed more structure, not less. Doing a bit of a Lifestyle Audit for *every* woman, I determined that there are really only seven different options for personal Youniform types.

If the lifestyle audit left you feeling a bit hazy, then the 7 Foolproof Outfits will give you the clarity you need to keep moving forward.

Our lives are a tapestry of interactions—from professional to personal, they can be grouped by intent and dress code for most purposes. While there's always plenty of variety from one woman to the next, the hierarchy of situational dressing remains the same. The 7 Foolproof Outfits provides a way of grouping the lifestyle activities into done-for-you arrangements so you can clearly identify which ones are appropriate for your life today, and make specific choices about what you need to fill each Youniform.

I'd like to tell you that I carefully made notes to develop this framework, but it was more of an *aha* moment after years of helping clients wade through their lifestyle audits and get stuck. In its full glory, it includes spreadsheet planning to account for seasonal variations and takes a few liberties with the 4-Piece Wardrobe, while also including some oft-forgotten accessories (cozy relaxing blanket anyone?) to carefully cover all your style needs.

Just like it sounds, 7 Foolproof Outfits is my gift of the Lifestyle Audit tailored to any potential dressing need and includes the following categories:

1. Casual at Home

2. Work/Professional

3. Community Casual

4. Going Out

5. Loungewear

6. Activities/Hobbies

7. Dresses

Each one comes with its own little quirks, and below you'll see how each one works with a full wardrobe.

Before covering each outfit concept, it's worth noting that three to five categories still seem to be the sweet spot for most women. Maybe it's because there are only so many hours in the day, or because we naturally gravitate toward similar lifestyle events, but there's no rule that says you have to fill them all. Use this planning tool alongside your lifestyle audit to easily clarify your own Youniform needs. As you read through each category, simply place a checkmark next to the ones that match your current lifestyle demands. Most busy women discover they need only three or four categories at most.

Casual at Home

The *Casual at Home* outfit is fairly popular with many of my clients, as it covers a wide range of needs. From the stay at home mom to the retiree to the work from home entrepreneur, this is often the workhorse outfit of those who don't have an office job.

This outfit ensures that you are fully dressed, even if you're not leaving the house.

2020 is still close enough that we all remember the lockdowns. "Stay home to stop the spread,"... but it didn't stop the spread of choosing pajamas, athletic wear, or loungewear as the default clothing style.

The idea that there's no reason to get dressed doesn't mean there's actually no reason to get dressed. Most of us live with other people, and they deserve to see that we think being with them is important enough to make some effort. But even if you live alone, you and your reflection are important enough to get dressed your best (for the situation).

Things to avoid: loungewear or pajamas (separate category), wearing old stained clothes because you're afraid to get the nice ones dirty (apron my friend), pants that are uncomfortable if you sit down for very long, skipping a bra and/or shoes (studies show getting fully dressed increases productivity).

Work & Professional

The next outfit is *Work/Professional*, and for many people this is a no-brainer category. If you have a job outside the home, you know what you need to wear to work. For many people there's an actual required uniform for this category, but for the rest, creating a fun Youniform is the next best thing.

From business professional to casual Fridays to manual labor jobs, duplicating your workwear is highly impactful and grants you more decision-making in your day. Don't be afraid to expand this category beyond the 4-Piece Wardrobe to ensure you simplify your laundry needs.

Things to avoid: having more than 2-3 work Youniforms, ignoring social expectations around what is appropriate for your career and title, a lack of color variety (unless you are required to wear a certain color on repeat), shoes that hurt your feet.

Community Casual

Community Casual is similar to the *Casual at Home*, and many of the same thoughts apply. Some of my more formal clients choose the community version for being at home, while others separate the two.

This category is quite broad and could include things like coffee dates, informal meetings, religious gatherings, volunteer work, conferences, and the list goes on. The differentiating factor here is usually that at home we are dressing for ourselves and the tasks at hand, while in the community we are dressing up a bit more for social interaction.

For many women who are at home most of the time, adding a bit of pizazz to Community Casual gives them a taste of getting dolled up again, which always feels exciting.

Things to avoid: ripped or stained clothing (unless you're doing a Habitat for Humanity day, save the holes for home), dressing down to fit in (just be yourself), clothing that doesn't fit properly, showing off designer logos (wealth whispers - high quality doesn't need flashy symbols).

Going Out

If you're a millennial or Gen X, you know what a *Going Out* outfit means. For many of us, it brings back the hot girl club era, but the same principles of getting extra fancy apply here to this category. For many women, this could include date nights, girls' night out, theater or concert events. You might choose richer fabrics or a bit of sparkle for excitement. But this category is also a great place for those who need semi or formal options regularly. This Youniform might be a bit smaller depending on your schedule, but it is generally the most elevated and fancy look in your closet.

I was inspired to create this category after working with my client Vanessa. During the week, she lived in tailored blazers and polished slacks for her corporate job, but on date nights with her husband, she transformed into a vision of elegance in stunning strapless sheath dresses. Seeing that clear shift reminded me that every woman deserves a version of "going out" that fits her life now—not the one she left behind.

Things to avoid: collecting too many fancy items if you only go out once a month, defaulting to black (always choose flattering colors), clothes that could malfunction (no indecent exposures allowed), expensive items you will only wear once (choose rental).

Loungewear

The *Loungewear* outfit is near and dear to my heart, and that of many of my clients. It was born out of the reality that many of us are suffering with chronic illnesses or conditions and don't have the energy some days to put on "real clothes." Belinda is one of my long-standing clients and calls hers "not quite pajamas" and mentions that being intentional with clothing that is above sleepwear when she is struggling with autoimmune flares makes a tremendous difference on how she feels.

There's a powerful mental shift that happens between pajamas and loungewear, and even if you are resting on the sofa all day, you'll feel better if your clothing is intentional, cozy, and you're not embarrassed to open the door if someone knocks. Imagine this scenario: you are laid out with a migraine, and your lovely friend decides to surprise you with some homemade soup. This thoughtful gift is amazing, but the whole time, you're feeling embarrassed and ashamed because you're wearing the wrinkled, slept-in t-shirt and sweats that you call pajamas. What if instead, you had designated cozy clothes for those days, and you greeted her warmly knowing that even though you feel awful, you don't look it.

These clothes aren't intended to leave the house, but would still fit in if you had to. Ironically, this is the one outfit I work on the most with clients, as most struggle to find the sweet spot between actual pajamas and real clothes. But I strongly believe every woman should have a loungewear Youniform that makes her feel amazing for being lazy at home.

Things to avoid: uncomfortable fabrics and styles, buying actual pajamas and calling them loungewear (these are separate), using your loungewear as your casual at home option (get dressed when you can), having too little or not enough in this category.

Activities & Hobbies

An *Activity/Hobby* outfit is a specialized Youniform for activities that require something outside these other categories. Just like in the swimming/diving category from my grad school days, this could encompass a wide range from sports or fitness, to arts and crafts to gardening. Only you know what you need to make the most of this time of enjoyment and creativity, and I would encourage you to create clothing that is separate from your other Youniforms if needed.

Things to avoid: using pajamas for messy hobbies (pajamas are for sleeping), having a disproportionate quantity for your weekly needs (do you actually work out seven days a week or is it more like 4-5?), ignoring your best colors (neon yellow flatters very few), forgetting to include protective items like gloves or aprons.

Dresses

The final *Dresses* outfit is one that can experience crossover with many others. You could have a dress Youniform for either casual option, work, going out, and even loungewear. But as I illustrated with my own example, since a dress (or jumpsuit) is a one-piece item, it requires a bit of modification to the 4-Piece Wardrobe to be more functional. I'll admit my entire wardrobe is a collection of dress Youniforms: a core casual with variations for home versus community, a professional version for public-facing events, and a lounge version that's essentially an elevated mumu. Be sure to follow the guidelines for the specific category in which you are creating the dress-based Youniform.

Things to avoid: ignoring silhouette for comfort (pay attention to your personal line to find the most flattering cuts), having too few options to maximize the mix and match potential, thinking a dress is more work to wear (spoiler: it's actually just one item and easier), saving dresses for a special event versus wearing them every day.

Whether you are comfortable with the Lifestyle Audit or prefer the structure of the 7 Foolproof Outfits, these methods provide a system for expanding the concept of one great outfit into a closet filled with the perfect outfit for any occasion. Every day you get the privilege of getting dressed appropriately for what you have planned, and you get to experience the confidence of dressing for the life you have. You have become a well-dressed woman every minute of the day, from client meetings to kids' birthdays, having coffee with your bestie, and even looking glamorous with the flu (maybe a stretch).

Getting dressed no longer feels frustrating and overwhelming because you have a plan designed for your life today, and you're ready for anything. But what happens when you want to mix pieces between your different uniforms? That's where many women get confused, so let me clear that up for you.

Master Mix-and-Match Style with Zero Guesswork

With multiple outfit modules in play, the most common question I'm asked is whether or not the clothes can be mixed across them. The answer is a resounding yes.

One of the big selling points of a traditional capsule wardrobe is variety, specifically the ability to mix and match all the pieces together. Visually, I have found this to be a powerful selling point, but in practice this is rarely the case, and differing silhouettes is the reason why.

When we create Youniforms, we create full outfits that are designed to be flattering and then replicate the components. One thing to be considered is silhouette, as mentioned in a previous chapter. Silhouette refers to the shape of your body (personal) and the shape the clothing makes (clothing). In situations where an item doesn't seem to work with another, it usually comes down to this principle.

When we consider our various Youniforms, we can often mix and match pieces. Let's look at a few situations where this works well, and a few where it doesn't.

- ***Yes:* The Going Out Top**: You created a going out Youniform of designer jeans and dressy, fashion tops and your work Youniform is a pencil skirt, cashmere tee, and casual jacket. In this case, we can likely swap both directions: the dressy top could be worn with the skirt and the cashmere tee with the jeans.

- ***No:* The Lounge Tunic**: For relaxing at home you choose leggings and a tunic length sweater, and your casual at home is wide leg jeans and a basic crew neck tee. In this case swapping may not work: the tunic may be too wide for the jeans, and the tee with leggings might require a layer to cover your bum. Either of these is likely to throw off your silhouette.

- ***Yes:* The Pro Blazer:** You have a work Youniform that includes a hip length one button fitted blazer with pants and a top, and community casual is a simple sheath dress with cardigan. You can easily wear blazers with the dresses and the cardigans with your work pants if desired.

- ***No*: The Longline Cardigan:** You have a dress Youniform that uses a wider swing dress with sandals for those hot summer months, and a casual at home Youniform with skinny jeans, tee, and long waterfall cardigan. The pieces here are going to be difficult to mix. Wearing the tee over the dress can be done but you have to "hack" the styling (tying a knot for example), which can look messy. On the other hand, wearing the cardigan with the dress can make you look shapeless, which may be cozy for at home, but won't be super flattering. You can definitely mix these, but they likely won't follow your personal silhouette.

Remember that the reason we can easily mix across Youniform modules is because of the intense focus on color at the beginning. Unlike a black/white/beige capsule that works because of a *lack* of color, the Youniform concept holds *because* of color. We'll be going deeper on this more in the coming chapters.

For now, I want you to go to your closet and take two quick assessments. First, count how many items you have that are true workhorses that go with everything. Then, count the number of items you have that never seem to work with anything. Grab a piece of paper and jot down the exact numbers. Most women are surprised to find they have far more "never works" pieces than "goes with everything" ones. If your results look like most of my clients, you'll have three to five reliable workhorses and fifteen to twenty pieces that rarely get worn. This should give you a baseline of how well you're already able to mix and match your closet.

When you carefully design your wardrobe using the Youniform Framework, the pieces are all intentional. Mixing and matching is often possible, but you will run into some constraints related to how the clothing falls on your body. This is why each individual Youniform is built out using the 4-Piece Wardrobe, so that even if you can't wear a duster with a maxi because you get lost, you still have sixteen outfits for each of the pieces in their respective Youniform category.

Style Icons Who Rely on Signature Youniforms

It's tempting to look around at famous rich men who adopt a Youniform and assume it only works for men. The logistics I have already described, and there are many women who do this, as I can attest from reading comments in various groups about adopting a style Youniform. But this idea permeates even the highest echelons of the fashion industry, if you know where to look. We often think of fashion designers or magazine editors as the ultra-fashionable who never wear the same thing twice. However, there are a few women who show us that even the stylish woman knows the value of creating a signature look. After studying the wardrobes of dozens of highly successful women across industries, I've discovered that the most influential women often have signature looks that function as sophisticated uniforms. Here are three examples that might surprise you.

The first time I ever heard of Carolina Herrera was when I was working as a pharmacy tech at 18. My boss was a 50-year-old divorced man who drove a Corvette and liked really nice clothing. To be fair, he probably contributed to my love of nice things, but I remember he liked to wear Herrera cologne. Without a modern internet, I assumed that this must be a man.

In fact, Carolina Herrera is a famous female designer and has dressed several First Ladies of the United States, such as Jackie O, Laura Bush, Michelle Obama, and Melania Trump. As someone who landed on the Best Dressed List in 1972, you would expect her to have great style. Might it surprise you to know that she in fact has a Youniform: a white button-up shirt with various skirt styles.

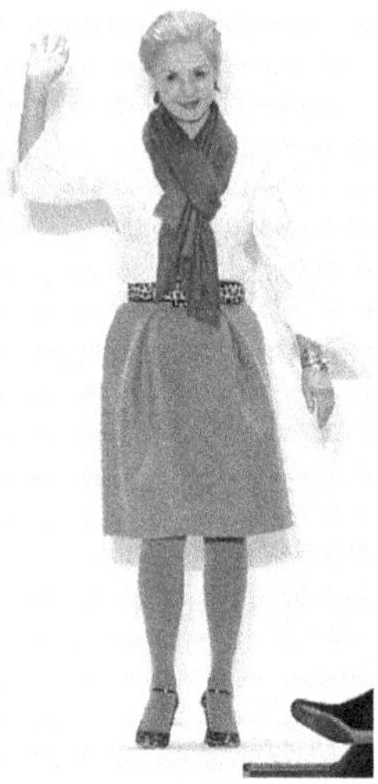

Figure 6.1 Carolina Herrera in signature Youniform.

There are dozens of images of her at different events all wearing this same outfit combo, from runway finales to red carpet events. When a famous fashion designer known for her great style chooses repeatable outfits, it signals to us that simplicity unlocks creativity and also creates a memorable experience when we interact with others.

Vogue magazine is easily considered the top shelf of style publications. I was personally never much of a fan because it seemed too out of reach, and those things weigh a ton. But even though my young-adult self preferred a good *Cosmopolitan* read, I always knew that *Vogue* is considered the GOAT. Paris, of course, pairs with it as the fashion capital of the world, sharing its status a bit with Milan and New York.

So what could be more top tier in the fashion world than being the editor-in-chief of *Vogue Paris?* Carine Roitfeld served in that role for over a decade and began her fashion career as a model. She was considered a muse in the late 1990s for design houses such as Gucci, Yves Saint-Laurent, Versace, and Calvin Klein. She was also featured on a best-dressed list, and, as you might guess, she also wears a Youniform.

Also, like Herrera, she chooses a skirt, always a pencil, with various tailored style tops to go with it. Again, we have a woman at the top of the fashion pyramid who consistently wears the same outfit on repeat, because she understands that style is found not in variety, but in being memorable.

But what of celebrities? It's common now to see them wearing new designers and adopting the latest street fashion as they flaunt their status or try to hide from the paparazzi.

But there's one that sticks to fairly simple and predictable outfits on repeat. Known for her iconic hairstyle on *Friends,* Jennifer Aniston is everyone's favorite girl-next-door to love. Although her Youniform is slightly less predictable, she typically opts for relaxed denim jeans or shorts, plus simple V-neck tees. Her red-carpet looks are stunning, but her everyday style is simple and repeatable combos, likely in high-quality designs.

As women, we often panic and worry that someone will remember the last time we wore an item, but if the most stylish women in the world can wear the same outfits on repeat, why can't we? We can take back the mental energy of choosing from too many options in the closet and make a swift decision based on our activity and what color we're in the mood to wear each day. We can feel confident in planned styles we know make us look and feel great, so that we can focus on the people around us and have meaningful connections. We can simplify our style and become timelessly elegant by putting together striking outfits that are just perfect for who we are today. And we can shop and spend and own less clothes while still enjoying quality fashion.

In the next chapter, we'll uncover the color secret that brings your entire Youniform wardrobe together.

Chapter Six Highlights

- Most women repeat the same few outfits because function and fit matter more than variety.
- A lifestyle audit reveals that our lives are repetitive by season, which means our wardrobes should be modular, not endless.
- The Youniform Framework expands one great outfit into multiple outfit modules that support real-life roles and rhythms.
- Most women only need three to five Youniforms to cover their current lifestyle without overbuying.
- The 7 Foolproof Outfits simplify decision-making by grouping activities into clear, practical wardrobe categories.
- When outfits are designed intentionally around color, silhouette, and purpose, getting dressed becomes effortless and confidence follows.

Part Three

Personal Style, Applied to You

"Color first! My tight color palette makes my Youniforms work even better. All summer with my knee I wore my skort Youniform or a dress, just a dress, because how simple yet pulled together is that? Both ways, I had access to a knee for PT.

"Pre-Stacey, I would have had many days in pj's, but getting dressed is EASY! Now that it's fall, I slid easily into cords/jeans and either a sweater or striped shirt + jacket. And of course, Keds!"

Becki

Seven

The Biggest Style Breakthrough

"While I know myself as a creation of God, I am also obligated to realize and remember that everyone else and everything else are also God's creation." - Maya Angelou

This is the story of how I finally understood that style wasn't just about the clothes on my body. It was reshaping me from the outside in, clarifying my frameworks, sharpening my focus, and helping me rise above the noise of style culture. I stopped reacting to what others thought and started anchoring myself in what truly made me feel authentic.

Something had settled inside of me by the end of my low-buy year. The simplification I had practiced on the outside had created the same clarity on the inside, and that alignment became the turning point in my entire style journey.

When my low-buy year ended I was a different person. The act of reframing my relationship with shopping and collecting clothes helped me learn to be content with what I already had. My headscarf fashion meant that I couldn't afford anymore to worry about what other people thought. The combination of those two things was powerful beyond words.

There were a dozen things that happened to me internally during that year that aren't relevant to this material. It was a period of massive personal growth, and I know it wouldn't have been possible if I were still obsessing over clothes, shopping, other people's opinions, influencer culture, and impulse buys.

My low-buy year ended in September, and my seventh baby was born in December. I made the self-care decision to take a full three months for maternity leave and delegated work to my team. During my first month of maternity leave, we had our highest revenue (to that point) period ever. Each month the growth continued while I spent time with my family, healed, and got to know my youngest daughter. I slept and ate and my brain started brainstorming again around the two-month mark, even as I kept resting.

What I didn't expect was how that same clarity would sharpen my eye as a stylist. When you stop second-guessing yourself, you can see solutions for others with a level of precision you didn't have before. The internal shift made my external expertise stronger, and my clients felt the difference immediately.

Suddenly I had reached the other side of this style journey, and I was actually experiencing the simplification that I had craved for over a decade. Building a closet of personal uniforms based just on dresses was unique for me, but it was exactly the thing I needed.

Changing my relationship with my clothes bled into everything else, and each part of my life became more intentional.

In this and the following chapters, I'll be sharing advanced strategies in each of the Five Stages of Style. These are the same steps we follow across all our programs to make Youniform building easy. Whether someone is in a DIY course, a group setting, or a 1:1 service, the process is identical. We return to these stages again and again because they create clarity every time.

The First Style Win Every Woman Needs

In 1923, someone asked George Mallory why he was keen to summit Mount Everest, and his simple response has become synonymous with the drive to conquer...

"Because it's there."

People have asked me a few times why I believe the foundation of great style begins with color, and my answer is similar:

"Because it works!"

Just as Mallory saw Everest as a challenge worth taking, color is the first challenge in style that's quickly achievable. It's the one powerful win at the beginning that transforms everything else and gives you the momentum to keep going.

Much like Everest is a fixed point, towering over the surrounding Himalayas, color is a fixed point in our style discovery. It takes some work to figure it out and get it right, but once mastered, it lasts a lifetime. But color goes beyond whatever the Pantone® Color of the Year is, or those colors that draw our attention in the store.

Color is an integral part of how we perceive the world. Everyone knows that grass is green, and the sky is blue. These are constructs we learn as very young children. Identifying colors comes early in the developmental process, and most of my kids had a favorite color by age three. Red is one of the first colors that a baby can see ("The Newborn Senses: Sight and Eye Color," n.d.), and often early infancy books will include this color on a black/white background because it is engaging.

Color is also a powerful form of communication. Color psychology is the study of how different colors convey meaning. People associate blue with reliability and trustworthiness, and red with passion and excitement. Each color family makes us think of certain things, and it gets even more varied when we shift how light or dark, bright or muted the color appears.

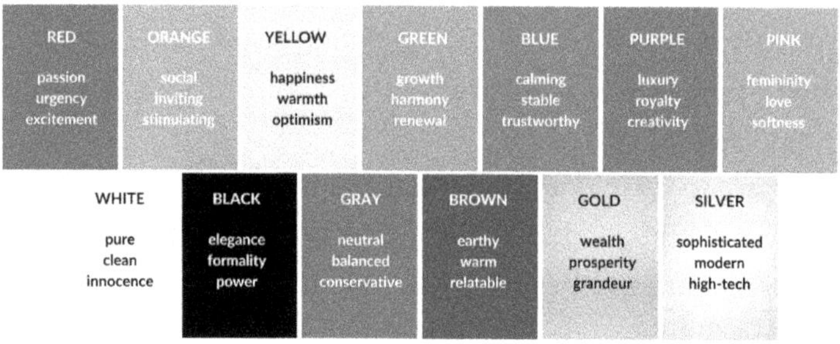

Figure 7.1 The psychology of color shows how different color families communicate (for full color images visit youniformbook.com)

For a woman carrying a to-do list a mile long, color becomes a way to control the energy of her day. The right colors lift your mood on hard mornings, give you confidence when you need it, and help you feel steady instead of second-guessing yourself. Color lets you influence both the room around you and the way you feel inside it.

But the best thing about color is that it's cohesive when applied to natural things. Color exists in many dimensions, some of which will be explained later. Each person has a specific sensitivity to color, and humans can see around one million colors on average (Pantone 2026). But every naturally occurring object is composed of colors that are congruent with each other.

When you think of a desert landscape, the color that often comes to mind is orange or brown. But when you deeply study that landscape, you'll see that the colors form relationships with each other that create a visually stunning experience. An image of the Sahara desert shows us the perfect color complements, as the waves of orange sand form a sharp contrast with a bright blue sky. An Arizona desert image provides a lesson in analogous colors as the tan mountains fade into green cactus, all set against a soft blue sky.

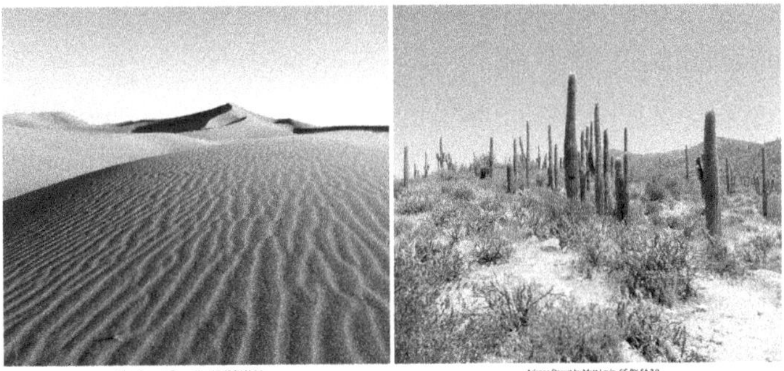

Sahara Desert by Thomas Woodtli, CC BY-SA 2.0.

Arizona Desert by Matt Lavin, CC BY-SA 2.0.

Figure 7.2 Two deserts displaying different colors in nature.

These perfect color combos are found in every part of the natural world, designed to provide a beautiful experience for us to enjoy. The macaw species of birds shows us high contrast in action, with the varieties of bright reds, greens, blue, and yellows displayed. Poison dart frogs come in bright, shocking shades to warn others that eating them is fatal. There's an old rhyme about snakes: "Red on black, venom lack; red on yellow, kill a fellow."

Humans fall into this order of creation as well, and each person has a color profile that is unique. Handed down from the generations before, DNA mixes to create unique color palettes that we can use in our style. Unfortunately, many of us don't see the power in our natural coloring, often wishing we had a different color hair or eyes. However, nature's cohesion proves everything perfect in its origin.

I didn't always appreciate my natural coloring. My best friend growing up had thick honey blonde hair, and there were plenty of moments I wished I looked more like her. I spent years dyeing my hair every shade imaginable: white blonde for a boyfriend, copper because I loved it, and burgundy after postpartum. I even pushed my fair skin too hard chasing a tan. Learning color theory finally helped me see that what I was born with wasn't a flaw. It's actually my advantage.

To truly understand how powerful our natural coloring can be, I'd like you to do a quick study of color in nature. Find three objects such as an animal, plant, landscape, etc. that occur naturally. Study the image of each object and ask yourself the following questions:

- What colors are naturally occurring?
- What is the quality of the colors (i.e., bright, soft, dark, light, etc).?
- Do any of the colors seem out of place?
- Does it seem like any color is missing that would complement the object?
- Why are you drawn to these particular colors?

Take just five minutes right now to do this exercise; it will shift how you see color forever.

When we can appreciate color in the natural world and see that it always works together to form beauty, we can apply this truth to ourselves. The color that we inherently have is also beautiful, and in the next section I'm going to show you how to hone in on those colors to make sure your clothes always amplify your natural coloring.

How to Identify Your Color Season With Confidence

"My mom always said I was an autumn..."

One of my clients, Denise, walked into her color session convinced she was an Autumn. She'd been told that years ago and had simply accepted it as fact.

She also told me that her best friend had claimed pink as her favorite color when they were seven, so she chose red simply because she needed something different. What she didn't know was that red was actually her best color.

In the 1980s a new phenomenon exploded on the scene. Women everywhere started asking "Have you had your colors done?" All this came after the release of the book *Color Me Beautiful* by Carole Jackson.

But color analysis actually has its roots nearly 50 years earlier with a woman named Suzanne Caygill. As a dressmaker and designer, she noticed that a person's natural coloring—specifically in their eyes, hair, and skin—correlated with the colors found in the four seasons of nature. She mixed this concept with personality to develop over sixty-four ways of categorizing individuals, by descriptor then by one of the Big Four Seasons: *Spring, Summer, Autumn,* and *Winter*.

When I first began doing color analysis, I was far too influenced by surface details like hair color. Experience changed that quickly. Working with hundreds of women taught me that color is not just what we see, but also how we express ourselves. Over time my analytical brain pulled apart every part of the seasonal system until I could put it back together in a way that made sense for real women with real lives.

When Carole Jackson brought this concept into the mainstream, she simplified it to just four seasons. In the four decades since, seasonal color analysis has experienced several iterations and further developments, and now is typically presented with twelve or sixteen variations on the Big Four Seasons concept.

At its core, color analysis is a style system based on color theory, or the idea that colors have individual attributes. This is the basis of stating that spring types are clear, or summer types are muted. The three aspects of color theory used in the modern system are hue, value, and chroma. Each of these combines to create a unique designator that describes your season with deeper nuance.

For most women, this is the first real framework they have ever had for choosing clothes instead of guessing and hoping for the best. Knowing your season creates clear boundaries that make everything easier. You never have to wonder why your friend looks incredible in olive, while it makes you look like you have the flu. You never have to worry about looking tired or washed out. Color becomes the starting point that brings joy and fun back into getting dressed.

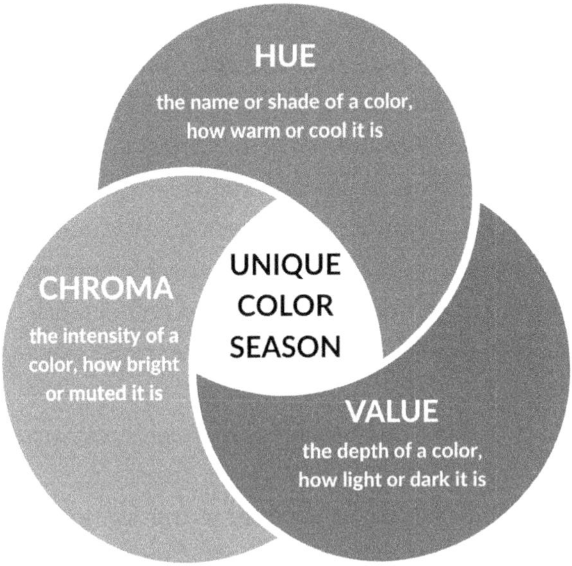

Figure 7.3 Color analysis is determined using hue, value, and chroma to find one's season.

When referring to color, hue is often a means of designating the color family: red, blue, etc. It is considered to be the purest form of color. In the realm of seasonal color analysis, this concept is greatly simplified into two categories: warm or cool. Analyzing the warm versus cool dichotomy is done in the eyes, hair, and skin, but it is of utmost importance when referring to the skin type.

The undertone of the skin is the biggest indicator of the overall Big Four Season, with the concept of neutral skin being a factor of having both an undertone *and* overtone. The undertone and overtone combine to form the external presentation of a more nuanced twelve or sixteen season type. Consider color mixing in primary school: blue plus yellow makes green. With skin we can see this applied to those with an olive complexion: blue undertone (cool) with a yellow overtone (warm) makes olive skin. Olive skin tones are always a cool type, usually a *Winter*.

The skin undertone is always red (warm) or blue (cool), and overtones come in a variety from pink to yellow, violet to colorless. Warm undertone types are *Spring* and *Autumn*, while cool undertone types are *Summer* and *Winter*.

With all these variations, it's no surprise that around 68% of the North American population is neutral...which confuses people even more! They get caught up in confusion about their base hue, just like olive-skinned people who often go years thinking they're warm-toned.

Understanding this principle simplifies color analysis and reduces the confusion over a borderline season.

The second color theory attribute to consider is that of value. This is how light or dark a color is. In color analysis, we use this to indicate depth in the eyes, hair, and skin. Although there are some outliers because of the third portion I'll discuss in a moment, typically those with light hair (blonde), fair skin, and light-colored eyes are usually a *Spring* or *Summer*, while those with dark hair, deep skin, and darker colored eyes are usually *Autumn or Winter*. For those with strong expressions of these ends of the spectrum, their value becomes a determining factor. For all the rest who fall in the middle, the last attribute of chroma often gives the season.

Chroma and saturation are different concepts in strict color theory, but for color analysis they mean the same thing: clarity. The extremes of this attribute in color analysis are bright versus muted.

In color theory terms, a bright color is a fully saturated color. A muted color is a tone—made by adding increasing amounts of gray to a specific hue. Clarity in color analysis can be a function of how the eyes and hair contrast against the skin, but it can also exist in the individual elements. A woman with naturally brilliant copper hair exhibits high chroma in just hair type, and may not have a high level of contrast with her skin. This is perhaps the most difficult attribute of color analysis for most to grasp. Highly saturated individuals are winter or spring, while low chroma types are summer or autumn.

Chroma is the area where most women get tripped up, especially when they cannot understand why black looks harsh on them or why certain muted colors seem to drain their face.

After completing hundreds of color analyses, I have found that the fastest way to read chroma correctly is to study the *eyes*.

Eye patterns reveal whether someone naturally belongs with brighter or more muted colors. Whether they are green, blue, or brown, eyes can be anything from muddy sage in appearance or bright blue with lots of patterning.

When you get chroma wrong, you either stand out in the wrong way or disappear altogether.

When you combine the three attributes of hue, value, and chroma, you could theoretically get twenty-seven season designations, but absolute neutral types do not exist; therefore those are discarded. When you put these together in a big picture, you get the following four color season types:

- ***Spring*** types are warm in undertone, and typically present with translucent, yellow, or pink overtones. The value falls in the range of ultra light to medium, and you see many light blondes and redheads in this type. The chroma for *Spring* is high contrast, at least medium-bright to bright. *Spring* shares an undertone with *Autumn*, but it is lighter and more contrasted. It shares value with *Summer*, but is bright and warm. Both *Spring* and *Winter* are bright, but *Spring* is warm.

- ***Summer*** types are cool in undertone, and typically present with pink, violet, or beige overtones. The value falls in the range of ultra light to medium, and cool blondes of various levels typically fall in this range, along with ashy brunettes. The chroma for *Summer* is low contrast, from moderate to very muted. *Summer* shares an undertone with *Winter*, but it is soft and light. It shares value with *Spring*, but is cool and muted. Both *Summer* and *Autumn* are soft, but *Summer* is cool.

- ***Autumn*** types are warm in undertone, and typically present with yellow, beige, or violet overtones. The value falls in the range of medium to very dark, but you do occasionally see rich blonde hair in this type. The chroma for *Autumn* is low contrast, from very muted to medium. *Autumn* shares an undertone with *Spring*, but is dark and rich. It shares value with *Winter*, but is muted and warm. Both *Autumn* and *Summer* are muted, but autumn is deeper.

- ***Winter*** types are cool in undertone, and typically present with yellow, violet, or pink overtones. The value falls in the range of medium to very dark, and it is rare to see pale hair in this type. The chroma for *Winter* is high contrast, from medium to ultra bright. *Winter* shares an undertone with *Summer*, but is clear and dark. It shares value with *Autumn*, but is cool and bright. Both *Winter* and *Spring* are high chroma, but *Winter* is icy cool.

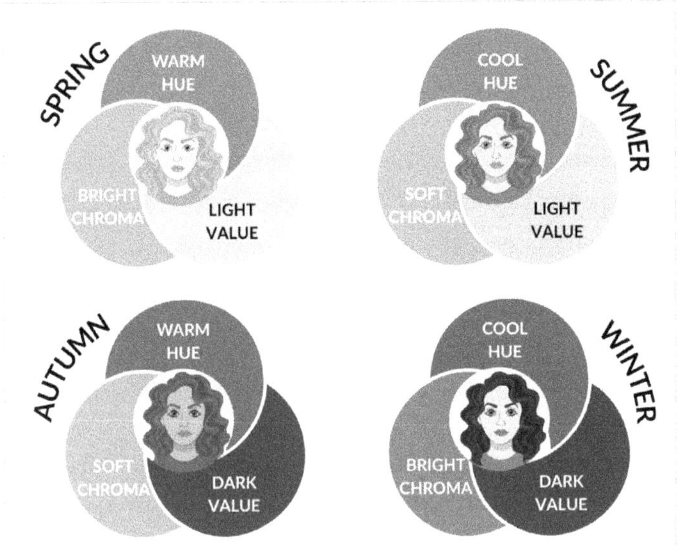
SPRING
WARM HUE
BRIGHT CHROMA
LIGHT VALUE
SUMMER
COOL HUE
SOFT CHROMA
LIGHT VALUE
AUTUMN
WARM HUE
SOFT CHROMA
DARK VALUE
WINTER
COOL HUE
BRIGHT CHROMA
DARK VALUE

Figure 7.4 Big Four Season color analysis showing hue, value, and chroma for each.

You do not need to master all of this. Start by noticing which season you feel drawn to, because that instinct is often your first clue. The real goal is understanding which colors make you feel alive, confident, and like the best version of yourself.

Now that you understand the basics of color theory and how it applies to color analysis to create four distinct seasons, I'd love for you to decide which one of these suits you best. Wearing colors that flatter your natural coloring can improve your appearance by at least 50%, even if you change nothing else about your style. Ask yourself these questions to get clarity:

- Do I have more of a blue undertone or red? You can study the color your cheeks flush as an indicator: pinkish plum means cool, coral red means warm.
- Are my features more light in value or dark? Light hair, skin, and eyes, or dark? Or are you somewhere in the middle?
- Are your features bright and striking? Do you have vivid eyes, richly colored natural hair, or luminescent skin? Or do they all blend together?

Give yourself three minutes in natural light to answer these questions. You will walk away with more insight about your coloring than most women ever receive.

Build Your Wardrobe With Just 11 Colors

Finding your color season is truly life changing and will give you the freedom to say yes to some colors and no to others. But you might also feel overwhelmed when you see the entire range of 30+ colors you can use. When my client Elizabeth first found her season, she admittedly went a little crazy. She started buying every single item she saw that was in her season. If it looked close enough, it jumped into her cart. She was so excited by this newfound confidence that she didn't stop to edit her choices. She later told me she ended up getting rid of most of it, because it wasn't even her style.

We can't stuff every conceivable color in our closet and hope for functionality.

I made the same mistake when I first learned I was a Winter. I bought every color in the palette because it all technically worked. Then I realized I had never enjoyed wearing red, and white was not practical for a mom with small kids. Trying to collect every color was actually creating more confusion. I needed to focus on the few colors I truly loved. It is completely normal to go overboard at first, but I want you to skip that step and start with the clarity of a wardrobe color palette.

When you think of a color palette, you might think about those handheld trays that artists use to hold their paint. That actually provides a great analogy for us:

Just like the painter can't use every single color in their painting and hope for something beautiful, we can't stuff every conceivable color in our closet and hope for functionality.

The artist knows to focus on specific colors, weaving them together in a way that creates harmony. Think of Monet's Water Lilies...you would see blue, green, yellow, white, and even red used to create that iconic painting.

Beautiful things do not happen by accident. Artists choose specific colors on purpose, and the same principle applies to your wardrobe. Women who live with intention do not leave their style to chance. Your closet needs the same thoughtful curation you give your daily planner. That is how you create a wardrobe that looks gorgeous, functions well, and actually mixes and matches.

The palette you create for your closet holds a variety of colors that work together to bring cohesion and beauty into your closet. A well-designed color palette becomes the North Star for your style, giving you a foundation to shop, declutter, build outfits, and more. It allows you to choose some colors to make prominent in your closet because you truly love them and they make you glow. No one is forcing you to wear colors you don't like. Your palette is intended to shift with you over time, even if you suddenly fall in love with a color you thought you hated, like my client Lana did with mauve.

Lana is a homeschooling entrepreneur who teaches journaling for personal growth. When we first worked on her palette, she told me she hated anything pink because it always felt too girly. I encouraged her to try a soft mauve, because it fit her Summer palette beautifully. The moment she put it on, everything lifted. She felt feminine and beautiful in a way that surprised her. Now mauve is one of her signature colors, and it is something we always look for when we do personal shopping sessions.

Once you know your season, your options become more limited, but this gives you a place to start building your own color palette with confidence. We always start with neutrals because they form a foundation of your style. Neutrals are colors like black, brown, beige, navy, white, ivory, etc., that should match any other color you put with them. Neutral colors should make up the core of your closet, and at any given time 50-70% of your clothes should be these color powerhouses.

When it comes to choosing neutral colors for a closet color palette, I recommend starting with four to give you a strong foundation. You should always choose a dark neutral, and for many this might be black, but if black is extremely unflattering and harsh, some common options are navy, charcoal, or espresso/chocolate. These are the most common non-black options (therefore easy to find), but any color taken to its darkest form can function as a black alternative. You should also choose a version of white for your color palette. Just like with your version of black, it needn't actually be white. Some other great choices here include soft white, ivory, or cream.

With our darkest and lightest neutrals chosen, it's time to talk about those two extra neutrals. One of them should be a mid-range color that works with the two you've chosen so far. For example, if black and white are your choices, a medium gray will make the most sense. If you've chosen chocolate and cream, then a beige will work well.

It's of note here that you'll often see neutral closets that contain black and beige; the truth is that those two colors don't work for someone in the same season 99.9% of the time, so don't feel like you need to make this work for you. I have seen this mistake so many times that I have named it the "sad beige aesthetic." Women buy black and beige because the internet calls them essentials, but black belongs to winters and beige belongs to spring and autumn types. For most women, forcing them together means half the closet ends up unflattering and wasted.

Your fourth and final neutral selection is a bit of a wildcard. You can put anything here that you think you'd like to wear. Many of my clients choose to put denim here, and the denim you choose should follow the value distinction of your season: Spring and Summer choose light to medium wash, Autumn and Winter choose medium to dark wash. For others, there might be an outlier common neutral like navy or beige that you want to add. For my clients that love a *lot* of color, they will often add something we lovingly refer to as a "color neutral"...colors that are commonly used as a neutral shade like olive, blush, or burgundy. This exists to give you a bit more variety in your closet. As a winter, my neutrals are black, white, charcoal, and navy. Go to **youniformbook.com** to see examples of client palettes and get a template to build your own.

The next step in creating your personal color palette is to designate signature colors. Signature colors are the ones that everyone associates with you, and they should make up 15-30% of your closet. Steve Jobs is the classic example of wearing a signature color. His was black.

Yours will be different, but the idea is the same. Choose the colors that make you feel unmistakably like yourself. Some women immediately know the first color to put in this set, but you might have to do some digging to discover your signature colors. Think about colors that have always drawn you in, maybe that's purple or teal or green. Study your color season and find versions that resonate with you. These are the colors to use as your signature colors.

The final type of colors to include on your personal palette are your accent colors. These usually make up 5–15% of your closet and act as small splashes of fun. There is no strict rule for choosing them, so here are a few ways my clients and I approach it. You can use the calendar method and choose a separate accent color for each of the four seasons: bright in Spring, light in Summer, rich in Fall, and dark in Winter.

Some clients use their accent colors to include shades they enjoy but are not their most flattering. For instance, my Deep Winter clients sometimes add a rich mustard yellow in small doses because it makes them happy. Other clients prefer an ultra-minimalist approach and skip accent colors entirely. Four neutrals and three signature colors already create a strong, cohesive palette, so do not feel like you have to include accents if that is not your style.

Ultimately, your color palette is intended to be a foundational tool to creating a closet you love, filled with colors that make you look stunning. The colors you choose to put there should reflect who you are (more on that later), and make you feel excited to get dressed. When you look at a closet created using a color palette, you'll notice that it's not a rainbow, but rather a curated collection of mix and match pieces that give you tons of variety.

Creating your color palette is powerful. It provides natural boundaries to what you choose to keep in your closet. It is the foundation of building a Youniform wardrobe that mixes and matches and functions as intended. I'd love for you to use the free template and start now by creating your own. Visit **youniformbook.com** to access your downloads.

Chapter Seven Highlights

- Style clarity begins with color because it is a fixed attribute that does not change with trends, weight, or life stage.
- Seasonal color analysis is based on three measurable attributes—hue, value, and chroma—that determine which colors harmonize with your natural coloring.
- Correct color choices improve appearance immediately by increasing contrast, brightness, and visual balance without changing silhouette or fit.
- Knowing your season creates boundaries that reduce decision fatigue by eliminating colors that will never work for you.
- A functional wardrobe does not require every color in your season; it requires a controlled personal color palette.
- A wardrobe color palette is built by selecting four core neutrals, followed by signature colors that define your visual identity.
- Using a consistent color palette across all Youniforms ensures that outfits mix easily and support repeatable dressing systems.

Eight

Embrace the Real You

"Authenticity is the daily practice of letting go of who we think we're supposed to be and embracing who we are." - Brené Brown

When I completed my stylist training, we were given a textbook that had a chapter on different style types. The idea—of course—is that by categorizing our style we can more easily choose the clothes that flatter. But I find the standard way of using six style types to be sorely lacking. Often, women just choose a word they think fits, but don't understand how or why to use it.

I did this when I first started teaching clients and even labeled myself as a whimsical classic (what does that even mean??). Also worth noting is that I have a love/hate relationship with blazers, a cornerstone of classic styling. But beyond this level of confusion, the meaning of these words change over time and are subject to interpretation, so you can never actually be sure what your style type is supposed to be.

Take, for instance, the modern usage of the word "preppy." When I was younger, this term referred to polos and Eastern Seaboard-inspired old money looks. The 21st century version of preppy has merged into bright colors and bold patterns that read anything but.

Vague words and style types are really just boxes that we try to fit into to describe who we think we are.

You find authenticity in your clothes when you take your God-given qualities, both internal and external, and honor them in your style choices.

In this chapter, I'm going to introduce the idea of identifying your intrinsic style personality using essence-based discovery. Once you've unlocked this way of looking at who you genuinely are, your clothing choices will feel like a natural extension of yourself. By the end of this chapter, you'll create your own Essence Map—a simple blueprint that removes decision fatigue and gives you a consistent way to choose outfits that feel like *you*. This is the same process we use with our clients that consistently makes them feel truly seen for the first time.

The Message You're Sending Without Saying a Word

No one tells you that as a business owner, you're going to wear fifty hats and learn a dozen skills you never expected. Even with most of an MBA under my belt, I still find the sheer range of tasks overwhelming at times. Marketing has always been the hardest for me. Fun fact: I once worked as a telephone sales rep for a photography studio and flunked out after one week. Selling has never been my strength, but the world of marketing introduced me to one idea that changed everything: branding.

Branding is the way a business (or person) builds an identity that others can recognize. We often see this expressed through colors, logos, taglines, marketing tactics, and product design. When we choose brands, we rarely think about all the effort that goes into influencing our perception of their product versus a similar product. Why, for instance, does a person choose Coca-Cola over Pepsi? Why are some people diehard fans of Nike while others choose Adidas? It's likely because the identity of the brand sparks something within our own identity, and therefore we choose to align ourselves with that brand over another.

When I was a teen in the 90s, we would meet up with friends at the mall, which was the only place in town where you could find Chick-fil-A. At the time, their nuggets were amazing as an occasional treat, because their recipe and concept was unique compared to McDonald's or Burger King nuggets. I remember when their cow campaign started and the funny, quirky attempts to encourage people to "Eat Mor Chikin". In graduate school, one of my project partners was the owner of the local franchise, and I remember learning a great deal more about the company, like their low franchise fee and promoting-from-the-inside culture.

Now we often equate Chick-fil-A with Christian values, friendly service, ultra-efficient drive-thrus, and the original breaded chicken. Whether you love them or hate them, they have created a strong brand identity that stands apart from the local culture where they plant new restaurants.

If branding is an attempt to affect how others perceive you, then personal branding takes these same concepts and applies them to our self-expression. What thoughts do you think when you get dressed every day? Depending on the situation, you might think about looking nice to impress someone or being comfortable for a lazy day off. You might consider whether your clothes are appropriate for the occasion, or if you'll be over or underdressed.

You may never have analyzed why you're getting dressed, but each day when you choose what to wear, you are communicating with the world about who you are, what you believe, and how you view the world.

When you look like everyone else, who you are completely disappears.

And since every day you are communicating these powerful ideas, shouldn't you be absolutely sure that what you're saying is *who you really are*?

The problem is that most women never even get the chance to answer that question. Traditional style systems push them toward trends and categories that weren't designed with their individuality in mind. Instead of helping you uncover your true expression, they guide you toward whatever is popular, expected, or easy to copy.

But that's not always the case when it comes to our personal style. A few years ago, the plaid shacket was extremely popular. So much so that there was a meme near the holidays about everyone coming back into town, going out for a drink, and all wearing the same matching tan plaid shacket.

This is what happens with style: it begins as a trend, then trickles down until it's everywhere you look.

When you look like everyone else, who you are completely disappears.

In an effort to "fit in," we lose track of our own unique sense of self and style.

But when you take back your expression of style, you get to become the most authentic version of yourself and allow other people to really see you. Your personal brand strengthens because you become memorable, and your clothing shares hints about who you are: creative vs. quiet, colorful vs. neutral, edgy vs. timeless.

Then, you embody your style, which reflects your inner being. Every time you show up in the same style that is unique against the prevailing culture, people recognize something different about you. Your personal style becomes memorable, and others recognize it as your signature.

Maybe you always wear red, or you adore leopard print, or you always wear black jeans. Whatever your style becomes, it's an external expression of who you are. It's not subject to trends or whims, but instead is a well thought out decision about who you are and who you want to be.

But before you can dress yourself as a powerful personal brand, you have to explore what that looks like for you. Consider these six questions to develop your own personal brand statement:

- What five adjectives describe your personality?
- What are your strengths and skills?
- What do people think when they think of you? (3-5 words)
- What are you passionate about? Hobbies, interests, etc.?
- What do you do? How does it affect others or add value?
- Who do you identify with? (Real or fictional)

As you dig into who you really are, your values, personality, strengths and weakness, goals and associations, you get the privilege of exploring style in a bold way that most people are afraid to try. Instead of living your life wearing the same shacket as everyone on your block, you get to dress yourself in a way that is fully authentic and aligned with the person you are today.

How to Find Your Unique Style Through Essence Mapping

What I'm about to share with you is the secret to building a wardrobe based on who you are at the very core. Many wrongly believe that defining your style involves simply picking a traditional style label like Classic, Dramatic, Elegant, Natural, Romantic, or Sporty, and sticking to it. But what if I told you that your authentic style has always been there, just waiting for you to uncover it?

I remember the first time I took one of those "What's my style type?" quizzes. I checked some boxes based on what I liked for about ten questions, then the answer showed me their five style types ranked. I ended up as a whimsical classic, which is vague. There are hundreds of these types of quick discovery tools available, but with differing definitions of what "classic" means, they just end up adding to your confusion about what personal style means for you.

Enter Kitchener essences. This is a style theory that is typically attributed to John Kitchener, although it finds its roots in another creator, Harriet McJimsey, from earlier in the 20th century. Style Essence is a concept that goes beyond fashion trends and superficial appearances. It's about understanding the core aspects of your facial structure and personality, and how these elements are reflected in your clothing choices. Your style essence captures the true you...your inherent characteristics, preferences, and the vibe you naturally exude.

To further understand style essences, it's helpful to look at the concept of Yin and Yang, which we refer to as Soft and Strong. This concept, rooted in ancient Chinese philosophy, represents the idea of opposites and how they complement each other. In the context of style essence, Yin and Yang can help you identify the balance of soft and strong elements in your personal style. The Seven pure Style Essence types are as follows:

- **Dramatic**: characterized by its striking beauty and bold, contrasting features. Individuals with this essence often have a theatrical appearance that commands attention and exudes confidence. Pure Strong.

- **Gamine**: characterized by its playful beauty and bold, contrasting features. Individuals with this essence have a compact look, and their clothing choices often include bright, staccato pieces. Petite Strong

- **Natural**: embodies a casual, laid-back strength, often referred to as "girl next door" beauty. Individuals with this essence have balanced and even coloring, and their look is characterized by long, flowing lines. Softest Strong

- **Classic**: an even mix of strong and soft qualities, characterized by symmetrical beauty and balanced, even coloring. Individuals with this essence possess a timeless look, favoring elegant and structured clothing. Perfectly balanced Soft & Strong

- **Romantic**: lush and extravagant, characterized by sensual beauty and soft, sultry coloring. Individuals with this essence have a naturally sexy look, favoring clothing that is soft and fitted. Strongest Soft

- **Ingenue**: characterized by a small, tiny softness and an innocent beauty. Individuals with this essence have blended, flowing coloring and a naturally cute look. Petite Soft

- **Ethereal**: characterized by a soft quality that moves towards strong, embodying an otherworldly beauty with luminous coloring. Individuals with this essence have a naturally mystical look. Pure Soft

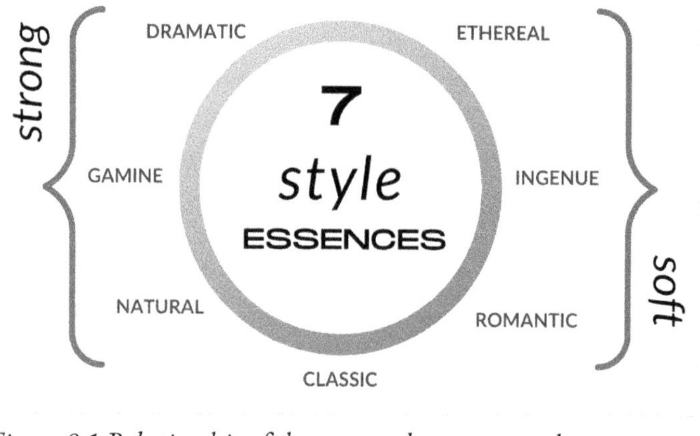

Figure 8.1 Relationship of the seven style essences on the spectrum of soft and strong (for full color images visit youniformbook.com)

The real power of style essence, however, comes not from having a single or pure essence (I've never seen this), but by the combination of several of them into a unique *style blend*.

As you put together 2-3 essences, the combination becomes something new and original, with the pure qualities melding together and building an entirely new style persona. The beautiful part of this process is that you don't *choose* a style essence blend...rather it's already part of who you are, and how you naturally express yourself. Many people suggest shooting in the dark to discover your style blend, but I have developed a process that considers the role essences play to create a full Essence Map.

This process has become the most groundbreaking key for our clients to uncover their style in every situation, building confidence even in those who have worked with stylists in the past.

Here are the components of the Essence Map so you can consider how these seven archetypes fit into your own expression:

- **Core Essence:** The strongest and most authentic expression; the primary style anchor. This is the essence found in your facial bone structure, and even if you do not like to express it purely, it finds its way into your personal style.

- **Flow Essence**: Naturally complements the core, making it easy to integrate. This essence is your preferred style expression. When you combine it with your Core, it creates a powerful synergy.

- **Thread Essence:** A subtle, underlying influence that is always present but not actively styled. This one often peeks out in unexpected ways like mannerism or facial expressions and can be integrated in small style details.

These first three make up your Essence Triad, and where you will likely choose styles most of the time. In other situations, you may find that expanding your Triad into an Essence Center is helpful for lifestyle adjustments.

- **Cozy Essence:** Brings comfort, ease, and a relaxed approach to style. For many people this will be Natural or Ethereal if not in their Triad, but any essence can go here if it makes sense in the way that you wear relaxed outfits.

- **Luxe Essence**: Elevates and refines for dressier, more polished occasions. When we get dressed up, we often choose styles that we wouldn't normally wear, and this part of the map acknowledges our more formal lean.

Finally, I have found it highly useful to incorporate all seven of the essences into a full picture of how we interact with each one. Therefore there are two outlier sections of the Essence Map:

- **Dream Essence**: Intriguing and aspirational but difficult to integrate authentically. This is your "it's lovely but I struggle to wear this one."

- **Anti Essence:** Feels least aligned and least like the individual's natural style. This is the one that when you read the above description, you immediately reacted with "nope, no way, not in a million years."

I used to teach small blends of 2-3 essences, but when my clients started experimenting with these concepts, I found several that had small bits of four or five essences. I wanted to explore how we could take this great theory and make it into a personal and useful expression of style.

Ultimately, Style Essence is a mirror reflection of what is already there: *You don't have to contrive to be something you are not.* And this sets you free to express yourself in your God-given beauty, which leads to massive confidence, more beauty, and more authenticity in your life.

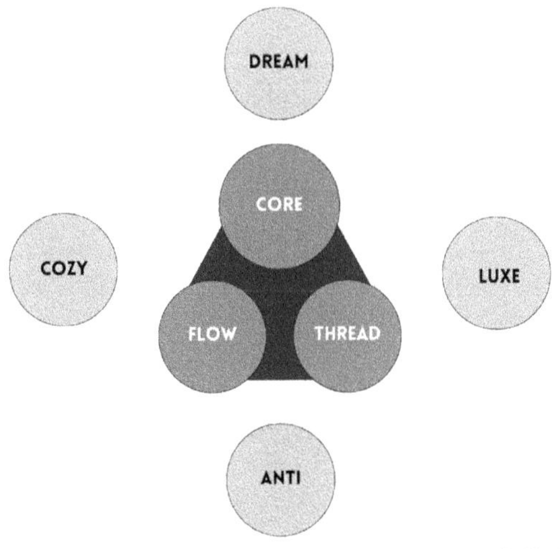

Figure 8.2 Diagram of Personal Essence Map™ to show potential relationships between essence types.

To begin exploring your own Essence Map, start with the Triad: Core, Flow, and Thread. Be mindful about the masculine and feminine characteristics of your bone structure (tough to be objective, so ask a friend), what essence you naturally prefer, and what other essence likes to peek out in small ways. Then check our extensive articles at Radiantly Dressed on each style essence to learn more about how to express your unique Essence Blend.

If you want the full picture of your complete style type, along with a full color analysis and starter Youniforms, consider choosing our ColorEssence Comprehensive Style Report. Learn more at **youniformbook.com**.

Creating the Perfect Style for Every Moment

In high school, my best friend and I used to share clothes. She would have the cutest stuff, and when I put it on, I felt like a lump of ugly. And there were some items of mine that I felt meh about, and she absolutely loved them. From the perspective of a stylist, I now understand that we have quite different essence blends, along with different color seasons, and that is why our closet sharing was mostly hit and miss.

One of the most crucial parts of advising others in their style journey is being objective about all the options, and not recommending clothes based on stylist preference. This is true for color seasons (some stylists skew results to their season, even though there is published data about seasonal distribution), and many people choose a stylist based on similar aesthetics. We often gravitate to people who look like us, but style is too unique to choose on bias. But there is beauty in every essence and every color season. The clients that also found beauty in all the essences was the catalyst for developing the Essence Mapping process.

In our group style program, we spend a lot of time breaking down outfits and identifying the different essence pieces. What is the print? What do the colors say? Which essence is a certain detail? What does the outfit say overall? It's the unique nature of the blends that creates something different with every outfit. Our clients repeatedly say this is the difference between being styled and *owning their style.* In daily life, most women gravitate toward their essence triad, or what is most comfortable. But the outlier essences can be incorporated into different situations in small ways.

I have a client (Client A) with a strong triad: Dramatic-Classic-Gamine. She is a perfectionist and had worked with multiple stylists and mentors over the years, yet her style never felt fully settled. Each analysis gave her pieces of the picture, but she was still searching for a complete explanation that felt accurate and trustworthy.

Before performing her style analysis, the Natural essence was a high contender in her primary blend. She leaned into jeans and leggings and sweatshirts and dressed the occasion for sporting events. All of these things find their home in the Natural essence. But when I looked at her bone structure and preferred outfits, it was clear that she was leaning into the Natural occasionally, but not using it as her main *wow* triad.

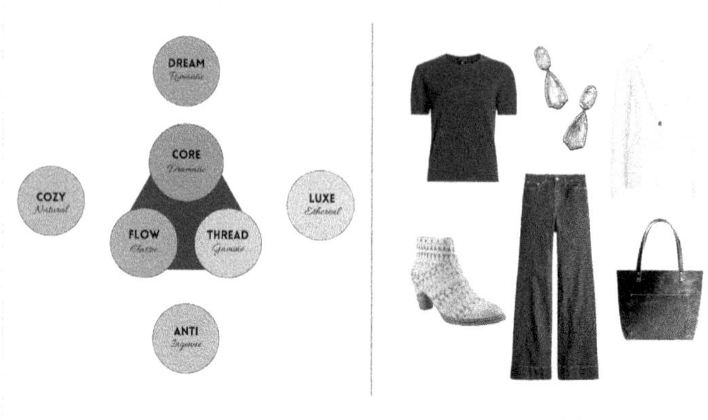

Figure 8.3 Dramatic-Classic-Gamine with example Youniform.

She also had a few outfits on the other end that were a bit fancy and outside the norm, where she leaned into her Luxe essence of Ethereal. The option of incorporating five essences becomes a powerful way to consider all the blend options. For her daily style, she can use Dramatic-Classic, Dramatic-Gamine, or Classic-Gamine. For cozy vibes, she can go with Dramatic-Natural (her preference), Classic-Natural, or even Gamine-Natural (less likely). When she needs to get dressed up, she can choose Dramatic-Ethereal, Classic-Ethereal, or Gamine-Ethereal. Each variation is a unique take on style, and she can let her mood and situation dictate what will look best and feel great.

After having many different style analyses, she said that this designation of Bold Autumn (see Appendix A for details) was the one that felt the most like home. This clarity brought an unexpected sense of relief. For the first time, she felt fully seen and understood, confident that her style finally had a name and a structure that matched who she actually was. Instead of continuing to search for the next answer, she experienced a sense of peace and confidence that allowed her to move forward with certainty.

Another client (Client B) was struggling with how to use the soft essences (Ethereal, Ingenue, and Romantic) and determining which one suited her best. With a definitive Classic core, finding the supporting essences was becoming confusing. Her report indicated that her triad was Classic-Ethereal-Ingenue, explaining that peek of youthfulness that was always prevalent in her style expression. With a very strong Classic core, she rarely leaned to Natural, but her love of barefoot shoes and natural fibers makes this her best cozy Essence. Her preference for magenta was explained by a Romantic Luxe essence.

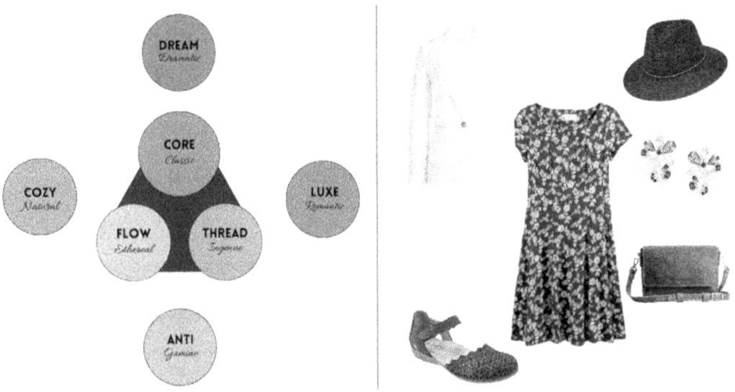

Figure 8.4 Classic-Ethereal-Ingenue client map with example Youniform.

Although she always chooses Classic and looks stunning in blazers and silk scarves, she can modify her look by adding either the Ethereal or Ingenue or both. But her options for blending include Classic-Ethereal, Classic-Ingenue, Ethereal-Ingenue, Classic-Natural, Ethereal-Natural,

Ingenue-Natural, Classic-Romantic, Ethereal-Romantic, and Ingenue-Romantic. Understanding the interplay between Ethereal and Ingenue gave her the clarity she needed to add the right delicate touch to her outfits. Instead of second-guessing every choice, she now gets dressed quickly and consistently looks more refined and aligned with her style.

There are twenty-one double-blended essences, which produces about forty-two major essence expressions, since the pairs can alternate which Essence is dominant. Minor essences can often be incorporated as well: patent leather for a Dramatic influence or a bobby pin for Ingenue. But the majority of any outfit can usually be described using a double-blend system. The power of the Essence Map is that you walk away with more than seven ideas of using essence blends in your style. If you mix this with the Youniform Framework of seven outfit types, you can experiment with your style quite a bit. Here is a sample breakdown of how each of these two clients might express their Essence Map through the Youniform Framework.

YOUNIFORM TYPE	CLIENT A (D-C-G-N-E)	CLIENT B (C-E-I-N-R)
CASUAL AT HOME	DRAMATIC-NATURAL	CLASSIC-INGENUE
WORK/PROFESSIONAL	DRAMATIC-CLASSIC	CLASSIC-ETHEREAL
COMMUNITY CASUAL	DRAMATIC-GAMINE	CLASSIC-ROMANTIC
GOING OUT	DRAMATIC-ETHEREAL	ETHEREAL-ROMANTIC
LOUNGE	CLASSIC-NATURAL	ETHEREAL-NATURAL
HOBBY	CLASSIC-GAMINE	INGENUE-NATURAL
DRESSES	CLASSIC-ETHEREAL	CLASSIC-NATURAL

Table 8.5 Table showing possible personal essence combinations for each of the seven Youniform types.

They could also just stick with the same essence core to keep it simple. The beauty of this system is that you get to choose dopamine dressing (clothes that make you feel happy) based on what you're doing, but also ensuring that every choice is fully aligned with who you were created to be.

When our clothes align with our intrinsic sense of self, it creates a powerful sense of familiarity when we interact with the world.

When you can get dressed in your best clothes in less than five minutes, you have more time to make an impact.

People are drawn to our authenticity, and we in turn get to affect more people. That's why integrating style essences into Youniforms creates so much clarity and simplifies your mornings.

When you can get dressed in your best clothes in less than five minutes, you have more time to make an impact.

Earlier you were encouraged to choose one Youniform type to begin brainstorming ideas. Now that you have learned about color and essence, it's time to think about which double essence blend might be the right choice for your first Youniform. When all the pieces come together, you can begin to imagine what a simple closet of twelve items in your best colors and unique essence can do for your mornings and your confidence.

But there's one final piece you need before your style can feel fully grounded: understanding the physical structure of your body. In the next chapter, we'll take everything you've uncovered so far and connect it to your body's natural lines and proportions.

This is the turning point where your style stops being theoretical and starts becoming unmistakably yours.

Chapter Eight Highlights

- Personal style becomes clear only when it is rooted in intrinsic qualities rather than vague labels, trends, or externally defined style types.
- Style essence is not something you choose aspirationally but something you uncover by observing natural structure, personality, and repeated preferences.
- The Essence Triad (Core, Flow, Thread) forms the primary framework for everyday style decisions and should guide most outfit choices.
- The extended Essence Map (Cozy, Luxe, Dream, Anti) provides context-based flexibility without compromising authenticity.
- Essence mapping shifts style from imitation to intention by giving structure to why certain outfits feel right and others feel forced.
- When essence is integrated with color and Youniforms, style decisions become faster, more consistent, and more aligned with personal identity.

Nine

Natural Bodies

"I've always found that beauty and confidence are synonymous. If you feel confident, that's what people see."—Cindy Crawford

I dislike pears...it's the grainy texture with every bite. I also find pitted fruits to be annoying to eat and cut, almost wasteful in both ways. I love the taste of pear, but not its texture. Apples, though, are a delight, both in texture and ease of eating. I hope you know where I'm going with this...

What would an exploration of style be without talking about body types? Our bodies are a source of both triumph and tragedy. Capable of birthing entirely new humans, and betraying us as we age with all kinds of breakdowns. From the top of our heads to the tips of our toes, and every piece in between, our bodies are constant companions on the journey of life. We rage at it, try to change it, and eventually (hopefully) make peace with it.

But when it comes to our style, our body is the frame on which all the clothes sit.

Throughout history, different body types have been in vogue, from rounded chubbiness during the Renaissance, to the waif-thin style of the 1990s. But the unfortunate part of this body trend cycle is that we actually have no control over the main shape of our body. Genetics gives us a combination of bone structure and flesh composition, and that's the end of the story.

Recently, I was hunting for a blazer for an upcoming photoshoot. I know blazers are difficult because of my narrow shoulders, large bust, and petite frame. But I took the blazer quest anyway with a reckless sense of abandon. I tried two, then reminded myself that I don't need a blazer in my life, and let it go. A previous version of me would have tried at least ten options before giving up, all the while blaming myself because my body isn't blazer ideal.

But if you hear nothing else from this chapter, your body is just a tool...meant to carry you from day to day. It's neither good nor bad, just a part of your life.

However, since everyone really likes to focus on body types and what works best for which type, I am going to indulge you with my take on body typing—a theory that is not my creation, but which I find beautifully aligns with my belief that every body type can look amazing.

Over the years, I've guided hundreds of women through this analysis, and one of my favorite moments is watching the acceptance and relief that settles in when they finally understand the body they've been fighting with. It's a shift that changes how they see themselves long before it changes what they wear.

What Traditional Body Typing Never Told You

We are going to immediately discard the five traditional body types: hourglass, pear, apple, inverted triangle, and rectangle. I taught this way back when I first launched the group style program. They were also in my stylist training, covered in a short, cursory chapter. I like to know (nearly) everything as I'm helping my clients, because I can draw information from my brain and help them get more clarity. Since my knowledge of the traditional system felt incomplete, I took a deep dive into it. For months I combed through books, blogs, stylist forums, old fashion archives, and every resource I could get my hands on, trying to map out the logic behind each recommendation. The more I studied, the clearer it became that the real patterns weren't in shapes at all, but in bone structure, proportions, and Yin-Yang balance.

I found theories and mathematical formulas for finding body shape, from hip to waist ratio to shoulder width. I watched the formulas break as clients who visually presented as one type adopted something else based on measurements. One tall client, who was obviously a rectangle, claimed she was an apple because of slight menopausal weight gain in the abdomen. The endless debates ensued over pear vs rectangle, and much of the published content overly describes inverted triangle as a "masculine" body type.

The deeper I dug into this idea of traditional body types, the more disgusted I became. They weren't helpful in giving women clarity about what looks best or mentally safe for creating body neutrality (more on that later). But the breaking point came when my brain assessed all the data and realized that every recommendation was based on one idea:

The hourglass is the only standard of beauty, and all other body types must hide their "problem" areas to look like the hourglass.

Rectangle? Create a waist so you can look like an hourglass.

Pear? Balance the top half so you can look like an hourglass.

Inverted triangle? Balance the bottom half so you can look like an hourglass.

Apple? Good luck. Wear a belt so you can look like an hourglass.

Hourglass? Congrats, you're perfect; don't wear baggy clothes.

I was done, finito, finished. My conversations about traditional body typing went from giving advice to ranting about the brokenness of that system.

Your body is just a tool to get you from one point to another. It's the thing that allows you to live your life fully.

What I eventually realized is that body typing—any body typing—is really just a cursory step in the larger process of acceptance. I still have women entering my world who are completely fixated on nailing their exact "type," convinced that if they just get it right, everything else will fall into place. But that mindset keeps them perpetually stuck. They're working on the surface layer while missing the deeper foundations that actually change how a woman gets dressed: her color harmony, her essence, and the Youniforms that simplify her daily life. Body typing can offer clarity, but it will never paint the full picture.

See, there's no "standard of beauty." We can sit and people-watch various couples to see that beauty truly is a personal perception and completely subjective most of the time. There's no need to become something you are not, just for the sake of satisfying a false idea of beauty.

So...we won't be doing that. Instead, I will present you with a new theory of body typing, one that recognizes the natural beauty and strength of your shape, and teaches you how to flaunt it. Whether it's commanding height or luscious curves, you get to be beautiful in your own right, no hourglasses required.

But since we're throwing this out, I want you to consider this—if you know your body type in the traditional system (ignore this if you don't, it's not needed)—what feelings have you had about it, both good and bad? Was it actually helpful, or just another way of putting yourself in a box?

And again, for those in the back, one more time...

Your body is just a tool to get you from one point to another. It's the thing that allows you to live your life fully.

It's just a body.

This One Thing is the Key to Dressing Your Body

Since I was a teen, I have wished to be tall. The doctors said it wouldn't happen, but with a mom that's 5ft 6 inches (165cm) and a dad over 6ft (180cm) I had hope. I stopped growing just shy of 5ft 2 in (155cm). Tall girl envy has been my life ever since. I talk to women all the time who wish their bodies were different: tall women wish to be short, busty women wish to be flat-chested, bottom curvy women wish they had breasts, thin narrow women wish for curves, and on and on.

I suspect the reason that we are all dissatisfied with our genetic body shape is because all body types have their own clothing fit issues. The small-chested woman has never had buttons gaping on her shirt, and the tall woman has never had to get her pants hemmed. We are all struggling with something when it comes to putting clothes on our bodies.

Unfortunately, I can't fix that for you. But I can offer you something even better: a new perspective on the way your body was made.

In 1987, David Kibbe published a book called *Metamorphosis,* which contained a new way of looking at style through the lens of body typing, called style identity. His book created quite a buzz, and he appeared on Oprah and other talk shows in the late 80s. In the 90s, it fell out of favor and the book went out of print.

The internet surge in the early 2010s brought his system back to life and created somewhat of a cult following. Groups and threads emerged dedicated to discussing his system. The growth of blogs and YouTube brought tons of commentary about his system...with the noticeable absence of David Kibbe.

Eventually, a Kibbe-authored Facebook group attempted to correct the public misinformation about his system, which ultimately led to his new book being published in 2025. You can still purchase the out of print *Metamorphosis* for several hundred dollars (I have copies of both books). I personally spent $300 for the original edition and invested several months studying Kibbe's updated framework so I could understand its strengths, its gaps, and how to apply the most useful pieces for my clients.

I have found using David Kibbe's concept to be hit and miss with my clients, who typically find style essence to be a better theory for embracing their unique sense of style. But there's a part of his work that we can strip out, which creates a profound shift in how we think about our bodies in relation to clothing and style.

At the heart of his method is a body type concept, which relies on five different types, each one demanding a type of *accommodation* for choosing styles.

Accommodation is an interesting word, and the definitions most suited to this use are: providing what is desired or needed, adaptation to adjustment, reconciliation of differences. Here, our different body types "need" certain types of clothes to look their best, we adapt or adjust our clothing to fit our body, and we reconcile that what looks good on a tall woman might not look as great on a short woman.

Each body type has one accommodation, based on specific indicators in the flesh and bones. These words also need definitions for this purpose. The bones in every body have a structural composition that is unique.

You may have heard terms like "big boned" but these aren't entirely inaccurate. Some people have a narrow, delicate bone structure reminiscent of the light airiness of birds, and others have sturdy, wide bones more similar to a carnivore. Neither is better, by the way. You can thank God and your genetics for the bones you were given.

Our flesh is a bit more complex to explain. We often think of weight gain as flesh or fat, but we can look at the morph body theory (ectomorph, endomorph, mesomorph) to see that flesh composition varies between squish and supple. For some people, they look muscular at any weight, but for others, the skin ripples and looks soft and doughy no matter how thin they are. But our flesh and bones make a difference in how our clothing fits and hangs.

The underlying Kibbe body types play off these nuances, and he will tell you it's not a body typing system. His updated book from 2025 is worth reading to better see how his system works. Hint: he also denies essence, but they are definitely integrated into his work.

Some might critique my take on adapting his system to be body type specific, but in working with clients, it's how I have seen it to be most useful. The following is my interpretation of his system, and how to use it to better understand the body you were gifted with. We will begin with the five accommodations, then move into how they can be combined.

Vertical accommodation

In Yin/Yang (soft/strong) principles, we would attribute this to the Yang end of the spectrum. People with this underlying body type are usually tall. Kibbe marks this at 5 ft 6in (165cm), but the limit used to be 5ft 8in (170cm). Vertical is seen in several places on the body, including the arms and legs, but also in the torso, as shoulder to fingertip length. One great indicator of this is measuring the space between your bottom rib and hip bone. Short humans like myself often have an inch or less, while my taller clients have reported up to 5 inches (12.5cm). Tall people do automatically have Vertical in their body, but this can also exist on shorter people in various ways: very short torso with long legs for their frame, or arms that end mid thigh on a petite frame (under 5ft 3in, 132.5cm).

Width accommodation

Perhaps the most misunderstood of Kibbe's concepts is that of Width. Width as an accommodation refers to the upper torso only. It's not width in the hips. But many equate Width with broad shoulders, and while it can be described that way, it's often a bit more subtle in its presentation. Sometimes clients don't have glaring Width, rather it is a whisper in experiences like needing to size up in shirts or jackets because they feel constricted through the chest. We can think of it as *openness* through the ribcage and shoulder area. Almost as if the bone structure creates the upper portion of an hourglass, rather than what we could think of as curvy breasts. Individuals with Width often have sturdier, thicker bones and have an overall athletic look to their frame.

Petite accommodation

For the purposes of Kibbe typing, we need to immediately discard our understanding of Petite in fashion as being someone who is shorter than 5ft 3in or 132cm. Petite here is more about the structure of the bones and a noticeable sense of narrowness. These are people who often look like they are stuck in the body of an adolescent, marked by smallness all over the body. Narrow hips, small sharp facial features, childlike hands, and feet. Many of these clients will report experiences of feeling like they are playing dress-up when they wear certain types of clothing. Getting mistaken for someone underage is another common occurrence. These types can typically go either way, presenting a boyish charm, or coming across as schoolgirlish.

Curve accommodation

I believe Kibbe overcomplicates this one as well, using language like "double curve" to create confusion when identifying this body type. Women who need Curve accommodation know they need Curve accommodation. If you've ever been grateful for those hidden buttons on a shirt, you likely have Curve. If you look like a sack of potatoes when you wear a swing dress, you likely have Curve. If you have to size up in pants for your hips but find the waist is too big, you *might* have Curve. Being bottom-curvy (what we might think of as a pear shape) without top Curve does not indicate that this is one of your accommodations. It is marked by extra curves at both the bust and hip, regardless of weight. I once lost a ton of weight and dropped to 95lb, and I still had a curved bust, and my hips did not get narrow. This is Curve.

Balance accommodation

Balance usually occurs in the middle of the system, but it's an accommodation of exclusion. Meaning, we have to understand the other types to get a full picture of needing Balance. Balance as a dominant type is the absence of all the other outliers. There is no pronounced verticality in the body, there is no obvious width in the torso, the bones are neither tiny nor sturdy, height is moderate, and there is no obvious curve. These things may exist in minimal doses, but above all else, a balanced body needs symmetrical proportions in styling: tailored fits, nothing too loose or fitted, lengths moderate and not extreme.

Now that you have an overview of the five body types extracted from David Kibbe's work, we can turn our attention to how the types can combine.

Because the system is based on Yin and Yang, Kibbe removed his "pure" types, stating that all people must lean either soft or strong. I think this also confuses the system when we can just focus on two accommodations and call it good.

First, you have to know and embrace your primary accommodation.

- Are you tall? Probably Vertical.
- Do you have broadness in your upper body? Likely Width.
- Are you small and narrow-framed? Consider Petite.
- Do your curves get in the way? Choose Curve.
- Do none of these resonate with you? Maybe it's Balance.

Once you have embraced one of these as your core accommodation, you may notice that your best outfits require you to consider one of the others.

- A woman with Vertical might notice she also has a wide torso, or is traditionally curvy.
- A woman with Width might notice extra verticality in the legs or arms, or curves along with her shoulders.
- A woman with Petite might realize she has very long arms and has random verticality, or she is blessed with ample curves on her small frame.
- A woman with Curves might be exceptionally tall, or very small, or she has to watch her proportions carefully.

- A woman with Balance might notice that she is taller or shorter than average, broader or narrower than average, or has a bit of extra curvature and need to adapt for that.

Ultimately, follow your primary accommodation in your body type, and consider what else needs to be part of your outfit. If this feels overwhelming, examine these five statements to see which best describes your experience:

- You are tall or have long limbs and struggle to find clothes that fit your length (Vertical)

- You often have to size up in jackets or structured tops because your shoulders feel constrained (Width)

- You have small delicate bones and struggle to find clothing that fits your small frame (Petite)

- Your bustline causes you to choose fabrics with give because otherwise clothing makes you look shapeless (Curve)

- None of these are really a major issue (Balance)

Identifying your intrinsic body type should be a joyful experience, liberating you from feeling like your body isn't good enough.

How to Accentuate the Body You Actually Have

Finding your primary body accommodation should have given you loads of clarity about the body God and genetics gave you. So now we turn our attention to learning to choose clothes that flatter the body you actually have. Before we dive into specifics, I want to point out that there are no hard and fast rules for choosing clothes for your body type. Those "rules" are the reason that traditional body typing fails.

Rather, there are a set of ideas to follow when it comes to choosing styles and shapes that work better than others for Vertical, Width, Petite, Curve, and Balance. Never think you can't wear something you love because of your body type. As you move through the next few pages, pay attention to the moments when something clicks or feels unexpectedly freeing. That's usually a sign that you're beginning to see your body with fresh eyes.

Another point worth noting...Identifying your intrinsic body type should be a joyful experience, liberating you from feeling like your body isn't good enough.

But many of my clients choose to use it as a secondary or tertiary method of styling, because they find their Essence Map to be more powerful for choosing clothing silhouettes they like. Remember that both systems are built upon the same concept of Yin/Yang (soft/strong) so any recommendation for Yang body types will typically also work for Yang essence types. In other words, a short woman with Dramatic-Romantic-Gamine essences and a Petite body type may find that she prefers wide-leg pants (Yang) versus skinny jeans (Yin). Keep in mind *all* of your style indicators to make the best choice for you.

I enjoy cooking and baking, even though the latter is challenging with multiple food sensitivities and allergies. My personal Pinterest is where I save tons of recipes, and I enjoy finding new foods to try. But have you ever noticed that if you google something like "blackberry cobbler" you get almost five million results? Now, none of us ever go past the first page of results before finding a recipe to try, but unique recipes have something in common with style: there are a million possible combinations. The good news is, you only have to find a handful of outfit combinations that work for you, and you can let the rest go (hello Youniforms!).

But this complexity is exactly why the only place I work with clients on body type and fit is inside my group coaching program, where we have the time and structure to go deep and address the minute elements of style that simply can't be covered in a single chapter. It's incredibly transformational when we can allow ourselves that space.

When you are designing each Youniform, consider all the specifics of each piece of clothing:

- What pant style do I like?
- What type of neckline do I prefer?
- What skirt silhouette looks best?
- Do I like fitted dresses or swing dresses?
- What length of cardigan should I choose?

Each decision you make is tied to your body accommodation and essence blend. Remember the five body accommodations as I give you some general guidelines for each clothing type, based on their Yin/Yang (soft/strong) applications.

Pants

This is where I always recommend starting, because once you get this part of any outfit correct, you have limits with the rest. I also know that women have a lot of fights with their pants regarding fit. When it comes to silhouette, pants do typically fall on a spectrum of soft versus strong. On the Yang/strong end of the spectrum, we see wide-leg styles like ultra-wide, trouser jeans, and flare legs. The volume and length of the pant mimic the strong structure of the body. Vertical types will like a longer line such as trouser or boot, while Width types may prefer the ultra-wide or flare.

On the other end, fitted pant types work well for the soft/Yin types. Skinny jeans, jeggings, slim fit are all great choices. These types can also pull off cropped pants better than the strong/Yang types, with narrow crops typically working better than wide crops (difficult for most because it mixes several types). In the middle of the pant silhouette spectrum are the straight-leg jeans, perfectly balanced, neither too wide nor too narrow. These work for most people, as other styling choices can pull them out of balance.

Skirts

These are another choice for bottoms, which I recommend deciding on before tops. Skirt shape plays a role here, but length becomes more important for the various body types. The Vertical types and some types with Width will need to be mindful in choosing midi or maxi length for skirts. Narrow styles like pencil can be good for Vertical, while those with Width aren't relegated to a specific shape (the upper body needs addressing more than the bottom here).

For those on the soft/Yin side, fitted skirts work well for illustrating the smallness of the bones, but skirts with some curved roundness also do well: tulip, godet, or flared. A-line skirts can be flattering on most, based on the amount of sweep and length. A full skirt, such as a circle skirt, often works best for those with extreme Yin or Yang (the volume of fabric creates drama that is held best by either Vertical structure or overwhelming Curve). Mini skirts are great for those with Petite body types, but Vertical body types can also wear them to show off the length of the legs.

Dresses

While there are many factors in what makes a dress work well, ultimately the silhouette should mimic the body silhouette. For this reason, dresses are almost always the easiest style choice, because the entire garment is one piece, and it either works or it doesn't. Sleeve choices and necklines also play a role, but fit must come first. For those with dominant Vertical, length matters, so choose midi or maxi, but also be mindful that the dress is sleek and smooth, like a sheath or column style. Width types do exceptionally well with swing dresses, since the shoulders carry the fabric the way it was designed to fall.

For Petite accommodation, the dress cannot overpower the body, but must honor the smallness: length ending at the knees and the upper body displayed like a fit and flare dress. If you have a Curved body type, do not hide your waistline (swing dresses are a no-no). Your rounded bustline will make anything unfitted look like a sack, and even a gorgeous sack doesn't do you any favors. Sheath, fit-and-flare, and wrap styles are all great for accentuating your natural waist.

For those with Balance, creating symmetry in your dress styles is the key, nothing too wide or too short, nor too long or too narrow. Simple, straight, somewhat fitted, a sheath dress is an easy option for this type.

Body confidence is self-confidence.

Tops

There are many styles of tops to consider for outfit selection, from tees to sweaters, they typically follow similar rules for fit by body accommodation and essence blend.

- Tees are tops that are typically knit fabric that drapes, but they often come in varying fabric weights. Silhouette and weight are the key. For Yang/strong types, choose heavier tees with boxier fits. For Yin/soft types, choose thinner tees with a more fitted shape.

- Blouses are a woven type of top that comes in an endless variety of styles. The structure usually means that they are best for Yang/strong types, but Yin/soft types can wear them with very specific soft and round details.

- Tunics can be woven or knit and are a shirt type that is longer than the hips but shorter than a dress. They require some type of undergarment like leggings or tights, which differentiates them from a dress. Woven tunics are typically best for Yang/strong types, while knit tunics work better for Yin/strong.

- Sweaters (pullovers/jumpers) are created by knitting fibers together to give heft and stretch. The density of the garment is key: Vertical and Yang can wear heavier knits like cable since their body structure can hold the weight. For Petite and Curve types, choose sleeker sweater styles that fit closely to the body. Balance can blend both: thinner sweater knits, but they can handle small, symmetrical cabling. Simplicity and quality work here; solid cashmere sweaters are a win.

Completer or Layering Pieces

Adding a third item to your outfit always makes it look more finished and intentional, and this is the hallmark of elevated style. These can be anything from a cardigan or blazer to a vest or jacket. Here are some general guidelines by type:

- Cardigans are sweater knit that are open at the front and may include closures like a zipper or buttons. In many ways, you can follow the guidelines for sweaters above. Length is also critical here: for Yang/strong types, choose mid-thigh or longer styles. For Yin/soft types, choose hip length or higher (yes, even cropped) to avoid overwhelming your frame.

- Blazers are a menswear-inspired piece that comes from traditional suiting. For this very reason, Yang/strong types do better with them as a whole. If you have Vertical or Width, have fun with blazer styling. For those with Balance, choose simple styles: single-breasted, hip-length, traditional plackets, and collar. If you are dressing a Yin/soft body type, you may struggle with blazers. Finding those with small details like a rounded collar or peplum fit can soften them up while retaining the blazer look.

- Jackets are a bit of a broad category, and include different styles like denim, bomber, puffer, and more. Visual weight matters here, with a puffer jacket working better for Yang/strong types simply because of their more substantial bone structure. Length is also a factor, and Vertical or Width types will choose longer styles, while Petite, Curve, and Balance should opt for hip or waist length. Given that these have natural structure, choosing rounded details for Petite and Curve can help.

- Vests also come in various styles, like jackets. Often if you get the style base (top and bottom or dress) correct for your body type, you have more leeway with these types of more unstructured layering pieces. When choosing a fitted vest like a waistcoat, follow the guidelines for blazers above. If your vest is essentially a jacket or sweater with the arms removed, follow those guidelines. For unique pieces like a flowy vest (or kimono) make sure that your base layer is on point for your body type, and adjust your lengths as described above so as to mimic the Yin/Yang of your frame.

These minor details are why putting together outfits can feel so hard. There are a million ways to put it all together, and some work best for specific body types or essences. If you've ever tried to copy an outfit and something felt horribly off, it's likely because the model had different characteristics than you. Understanding the nuances here is a heavy lift, I'm not going to lie.

My clients often spend months experimenting and noting the tiny details that make the difference between a ho-hum outfit and a wow outfit, which is why I stay with them so long. But anyone can learn this and apply it. Once you find your best fits, the Youniform encourages you to repeat what you know and save your sanity. My clients consistently report feeling more confident and excited to get dressed when they let go of all the clothes that don't suit them.

Begin today by examining your outfit using the guidelines above. Start with the bottoms, then tops, then layering piece and ask yourself:

- What pant silhouette is this and what body type/essence is it best for?
- What top style is this and what are the details? Does it fit my body type/essence?
- Does my layering piece follow the guidelines for my body type/essence?
- What changes could I make to the three parts of my outfit to make it more aligned with my God-given body?

There's one more activity you can do to get additional clarity on your outfits. Earlier in chapter four, I taught you how to do a body silhouette drawing. This is your personal best silhouette.

You can do a similar drawing of your clothing: take a picture following the same guidelines as before, and trace the outline of your outfit (vs your body). Compare the two drawings to see how similar or different the two silhouettes are. Your best outfits will closely follow your personal body silhouette. This creates harmony between your clothing and your body.

Making peace with the body you have is a powerful growth tool for becoming more confident *and* more fashionable. When you can accept that your flesh and bones are unique and demand to be framed for their beauty, you can let go of ridiculous body type standards that say only the hourglass is worth aspiring to.

Embrace your tall presence or your strong shoulders that hold clothes like a hanger. Love the curves that used to frustrate you. Or the small-framed body people compare to a twelve-year-old. Or the tummy that just never seems to go away. Or enjoy the symmetry of your body instead of bemoaning the fact that nothing stands out.

Every body type is beautiful and becomes even more so when we highlight the unique strengths of each. Release unhealthy standards of beauty and become gorgeous in your own skin. Others will see you more clearly, you will interact with the world with more confidence, and doing so will open doors to experiences that you never imagined.

Body confidence is self-confidence.

Make Friends with the Woman in the Mirror

In *Snow White*, the queen is beautiful in her own right, but so obsessed with her image that she constantly asks if she is still the most lovely. But we can never be the loveliest person in the world because beauty is subjective, and encompasses so much more than what the mirror shows. It's an impossible goal that leaves many of us feeling constantly inadequate.

Time marches on, so it's no surprise that one day, someone else is more beautiful. Fortunately for us, there's no magic mirror that tells us the exact moment our youthful vitality starts to fade. But that little piece of glass holds great power anyway.

When I was younger, my family used to make fun of me because I looked at myself in the mirror any chance I got. I realize how vain that sounds, and as an adult I can't tell you why I was so obsessed. Perhaps it's the strange memory from being twelve years old that set me on a path of admiring my face in the mirror. I was recovering from chickenpox, and my family had dinner plans to meet up with their friends. I suppose I *was* already pretty vain, because I had a large scab on my right cheek I deemed unseemly. Instead of waiting it out, I picked it off, and realized it left a huge divot on my face.

Stunned, I realized in the moment I had made a serious mistake and instinctively knew it would follow me forever. Resigned, I went to dinner self-conscious with a hole-y face. Midway through dinner, I overheard one of my parents' friends lean into my mom and say, 'She's so pretty, you're going to have to lock the door in a few years." Nevermind how weird it seems now for adults to comment on the attractiveness of a child—it was the 90's when weird body shaming peaked—but I must have internalized that compliment. And so, people often chastised me for looking in the mirror too much or for too long.

There have been times in my adult life when I haven't looked at myself in the mirror for days, and to be completely honest, I'm better off for it. Several years ago I listened to my clients talk about their own relationship with the mirror, and I was stunned to realize how many of them have extremely negative reactions to their reflection. Actual reports of crying when they looked at themselves fully clothed. In that moment, I embraced the idea of body neutrality as an answer to both extremes of self-image: body positivity versus self-loathing.

Body neutrality is a mindset of accepting your body as just a body, simply a vessel to get you through the day. It is neither good nor bad; it is just a body. It is neutral; it has no thoughts or opinions, and it doesn't act out (most of the time). Your body reflects your genetics and your lifestyle. One is completely out of your control, and the other is fully in your control. When you look at it, there is no place for worshipping it *or* hating it. It simply exists in various states throughout your life, the mortal flesh you are carrying around.

That's it. It's really that simple. But the body positivity movement would have you embody love for this temporal state. I would go so far as to say that body positivity is actually a toxic mindset.

Love the best parts of yourself, the things that make you truly beautiful as a person, and let the rest be like dust.

Imagine that you could get dressed, and check your reflection in the mirror, and feel satisfaction, but nothing greater or less. No self-deprecation or internal freakouts because your arms look fat or your hips are too big. You don't even think about the shape of your body because you are so focused on bigger things. You could walk past the mirror when you go to the bathroom, without looking to see if your hair is out of place or your wrinkled clothes make you look frumpy. You could even be so in tune with your body and comfortable that you could put on lipstick without using a mirror.

Body neutrality is about more than just the mindset part; it's about actually finding peace with the body that you have. Day after day, in every situation. For those with any kind of chronic illness, this may seem more difficult. I get this. I have been dealing with chronic hives for thirteen years, and when they are flaring up, I could easily default to blaming my body and thinking that it is broken. I could give up and admit defeat, resign myself to a life of pharmaceuticals to make it through the day. *Or*, I could accept that something has gone awry, making my body mad, and try to make positive changes that put them back in remission.

Whether it's our internal workings or the external flesh and bones, our approach to body struggles is grounded and healthy when we view our bodies as a neutral entity. Because the honest truth is that you will 100% have body struggles in your style journey. You cannot halt time, and it's coming for all of us. Whether it's the menopause belly, or sagging neck skin, or disability, or chronic disease, all of us have a body that is breaking down. I would always encourage you to make as many healthy decisions as you can to combat this, but at the end of the day, you can't stop it.

So you have to learn to roll with it, to continue to view your body as just a body, neither good nor bad, capable of great things, powerful in its own way, and worthy of carrying you throughout your life.

It does take time to reframe how you view your body, especially in a culture that is obsessed with youth and beauty. The prevalence of non surgical cosmetic procedures has sky-rocketed, with many women paying thousands of dollars for injectables. But when we don't have peace with our reflection, we are at war with ourselves. Just as the health of our body is a reflection of what we are putting into it, so is our self-image a construct of what we think about our body. If our thoughts are rotten, nothing we put on the outside will make us content.

I created a mini-course on body neutrality; it was one of the first things I made for my style coaching clients years ago. I'd love to share some journaling prompts with you to get you thinking about your body in a neutral, unbiased way.

- What are some body-positive statements you can reframe to make them body neutral? What does body neutrality mean to you? How would a neutral perspective on your body change the way you interact in daily life?

- What's your earliest experience where you felt like your appearance mattered? How old were you? What was the setting? Who was present? Did their words and actions drive your feelings, or is this memory based on internal thoughts?

- Stand in front of a mirror, study yourself, and jot down the first five thoughts that surface. Continue exploring why those were the things you thought about, both positive and negative. When you are done, choose three affirmations to stick on the glass as daily reminders of who you are.

- Name your inner mean girl and track her comments for three days, noting each trigger, the exact words she uses, and your initial reaction. For the most common trigger you uncovered, script three truthful comebacks that honor your body's purpose and strength.

- Write down three things you love about your body, and why you are proud of that. (Ex: my legs because they ran a marathon). Turn it into a letter praising the strength of utility of your body over its appearance.

I have often heard women say they are waiting for something to change in their bodies before they buy "better" clothes (for their style). But having seven babies in eleven years has taught me one truth: dress the body you have right now, because it will make you feel so much better.

And on the way to dressing the body you have now, make peace with it. It has served you well in the past; it has been a faithful companion, and it has probably caused you some distress, too! But that's just bodies. It's what they do. If we're lucky, it'll continue to do those things for many years to come. It is a part of you, but only a part doing its job.

A body is just a body.

You are already beautiful. You are "fearfully and wonderfully made" (Psalms 139:14, New King James Version). You weren't created to compare yourself to everyone else, but to embrace and express what makes you uniquely you.

Chapter Nine Highlights

- Traditional body typing fails because it treats the hourglass as the ideal instead of honoring natural variation in bone structure and flesh.
- Body typing is a secondary tool meant to support styling decisions, not a primary identity or measure of beauty.
- The five body accommodations (Vertical, Width, Petite, Curve, Balance) describe how clothing must be constructed to sit correctly on the body.
- Every woman has a primary body accommodation that should guide silhouette choices before considering trends or preferences.
- Body accommodations can combine, requiring outfits to address more than one structural need at the same time.
- Clothing works best when its silhouette mirrors the natural outline of the body rather than attempting to disguise it.
- Body neutrality is the foundation for confident dressing, allowing style choices to be practical, aligned, and free from self-judgment.

Ten

The Stylish Woman

"Everything has beauty, but not everyone sees it." - Confucius

My jeans sat in a drawer for two years. Long after I had adopted dresses as my daily style, I kept them stored away "just in case" ...What if I need them for a fall festival? What if I want to wear them on a super cold winter day? What if I change my mind and decide to be normal? But more and more time went on as they sat unused, and finally, one day after a client coaching call, I put them in the donate bin and never looked back.

I no longer own pants. It seems funny to say it that way—of course I own leggings for layering and loungewear. But dresses became my signature, go-to style.

I used to think that wearing a dress took more effort. I would look at the ones in my closet and never wear them because of the perceived extra work. I had ideas in my head about what the perfect capsule wardrobe looked like, and it contained multiple styles of pants, tops, sweaters, and maybe one dress...but it turned out that the reason I could never create the capsule I dreamed of is that I wasn't being true to myself.

I spent so much time trying to make clothes work that I didn't even like, just because someone else said I should. But when I finally stepped outside of expectations and gave myself permission to wear what brought me joy, my perspective on style shifted.

A capsule wardrobe promised me simplicity, and eventually I got there, but it was the complexity of the journey that granted me wisdom about who I am and who I wanted to be. The truth is that personal style is a journey into self-expression, with all its twists and turns along the way. And even when you think you've got it nailed down, something will eventually disrupt your carefully curated closet, and so you go back and tweak again—but each time with a greater appreciation for your innate sense of style, based on your actual life and needs.

My closet holds about sixty items now, most of which are dresses in various colors and patterns. I fully expect to get dressed each day in under two minutes, with the largest decision being what color or print I'm in the mood to wear each morning. Even on lazy or sick days, I have cozy dresses I can wear as my lounge Youniform.

It doesn't look like a capsule wardrobe, but it functions even better than one.

Every piece is tailored to the woman I am right now, and serves me as I go about my daily duties of raising my family and building an empire that encourages confidence and self-discovery.

This phase of the journey is all about style management and requires a few unique skills that we have yet to cover. In this chapter we will discuss the principles of shopping when your closet is mostly complete, how and why to declutter your closet regularly, and what to do if you find yourself in a life shift that has new wardrobe requirements.

The Power of a Master Shopping List

I really love to shop. My husband jokes that my solution to any problem is to throw money at it. I am also (quite humbly) exceptionally good at finding just the right item, knowing what words to use for searching, and helping my clients with those elusive unicorn pieces. In fact, being a stylist has done me a huge favor because it gives me an outlet for my urge to shop and collect, as I get to do it for others, and create gorgeous styles for visual platforms like Instagram or Pinterest.

I have found that there are typically two types of women when it comes to shopping: those that love it to the point of making it a hobby, and those who would happily wear an old shirt with holes to avoid it. I'd like to suggest something in the middle that helps the shopaholic rein it in and gets the naysayer curating mindfully.

I have always shopped for clothing with intention. My grandmother used to love to roam about stores looking at all the pretties, but I can recall marching into Mervyn's with a single-minded determination to find a pair of black slacks for work. Maybe I left the store with an extra blouse and some shoes (don't judge me), but every attempt at shopping started with one goal. Sometimes it was practical, and sometimes it was more frivolous (new dress for going out with friends). But always with a plan.

You are going to have to shop for clothes sometimes. And instead of being tempted by the aesthetically pleasing displays, or a random dopamine hit from a pink shirt, your shopping will be more beneficial to your entire closet when you do it *with intention*.

I am going to introduce you to an advanced method of curating your closet that works once you have dialed in your style and outlined your Youniform. I consider this to be under the umbrella of wardrobe management because, just like the Youniform, it has a process and a structure to make it useful without fluff.

Step 1

First, we begin with a list. But not just any wish list, or Amazon list, or permanently saved online cart (I see you).

When you created each Youniform module, you filled in specific types of clothes, from tops to bottoms and completer pieces. You did so following a very specific framework of two neutrals and two colors. You should have found obvious holes during this process; maybe you needed an extra neutral top, or a print cardigan. Maybe the idea of color pants was a revelation moment, and you put those on the immediate need list. You should have naturally been making a mental list of things you needed as you went through the process. But now it's time to organize those ideas into a way that makes sense.

You will create a master list. I prefer to do this in something like Google Sheets or Excel where you can add and manipulate the information. But paper works just as well in a pinch, as long as you can keep up with it. It doesn't have to be fancy, but across the top row you might add columns such as an item description, budget/price, notes, and which Youniform it's for.

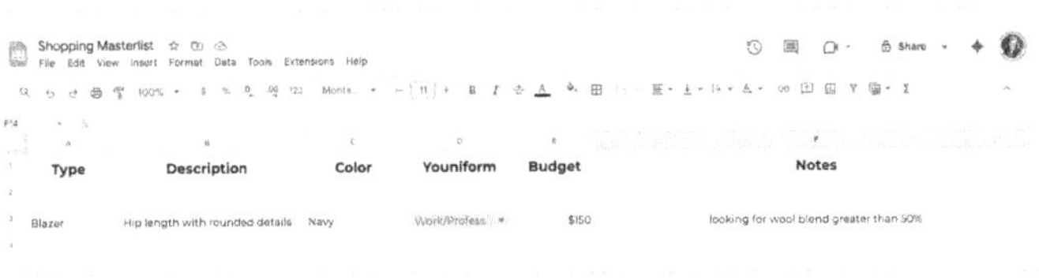
Shopping Masterlist
File Edit View Insert Format Data Tools Extensions Help
Share
Type
Description
Color
Youniform
Budget
Notes
Blazer
Hip length with rounded details
Navy
$150
looking for wool blend greater than 50%

Figure 10.1 Shopping master list created in spreadsheet format.

When you create it initially, dump all your ideas into it. Most people end up with 10-20 items at first, and you can add things here like jewelry, accessories, and shoes as well. Perhaps you realized you had nearly a full Youniform, but you were missing the perfect jewelry. Once you have emptied your mind of all your ideas, it's time to take stock and do some serious categorizing.

Step 2

This is where the list becomes your magic shopping secret. It's time to rank your list by what need is most pressing. Realistically, everyone will approach this differently, but some questions you can ask for clarity are:

- Which Youniform do I need the most right now?
- Am I missing something critical that would make a specific Youniform complete?
- Do I need something very basic for workhorse wear?
- Is there something I've fallen in love with and can't quit thinking about?
- Could this item potentially go out of stock and be unavailable if I wait?

The reason spreadsheet software works so well is that it's easy to move these around. As you are shifting, you should realize that there are a few things that you need/want more than the rest. You are going to focus on the top five for your upcoming shopping needs. The reason this is genius is threefold: it's based on priority and need, you acknowledge all the things you want without being overwhelmed, and you have freedom to grab anything in the top five.

As time goes by, clients get their closets dialed in tightly, with about a 95% near-perfection rating. But when you get to this part of the journey, your style has evolved to where you are ultra-specific about what you will allow in your Youniform closet. When this happens, your top five often includes "unicorn" pieces. Your desire for something is so unique and specific that it's difficult to find.

This is okay. Eventually the unicorn item will turn up, flowers will sing, and gold will fall from the sky. Not really, but it will feel that way to finally score that sought-after item. However, if that item was the first on your list, and you were laser-focused on it, you might miss out on items 2-5 in the meantime.

But with a top five priority, every time you go shopping, you are on the lookout for any of those items. When you find one, you move it off the wish list, and something below takes its place. Your list is ever evolving as you add one curated piece after the next.

Step 3

On top of the list, we can add another pro shopping practice to our style system. The 5-piece French wardrobe is a revolutionary way to approach ongoing closet curation. Again, this is an advanced practice for those who are almost fully satisfied with their closet and style and want to keep it fresh mindfully.

The premise of the 5-piece French wardrobe is that you shop only twice a year, once for spring/summer and again for fall/winter. Similar to the magic shopping list, you only buy five items. In between, you are considering and prioritizing what you want or need, and saving your money to buy high quality, long-lasting pieces. If you think you can't afford expensive, quality items, this process makes it possible.

The recommended clothing budget by financial experts is 2-7% of your income for the entire family. We can do a simple calculation on a family of four making $100k per year to see how that breaks down per person.

	2% BUDGET	5% BUDGET	7% BUDGET
ANNUAL	$500	$1250	$1750
BI-MONTHLY	$42	$104	$145
QUARTERLY	$125	$313	$435
MONTHLY	$250	$625	$875

Figure 10.2 Sample budget showing how clothing expenses are broken down for a family of 4.

This is simplified, because if your family of four includes two small children, their clothing budget is obviously smaller than that of an adult. Based on a modest 5% clothing budget and following the 5-piece French wardrobe, you can spend around $125 *per item* per person, which is plenty for quality clothing purchases. Even 2% goes much further if you spend it less often, making sure that you can invest in pieces that will last much longer.

This process of shopping less admittedly takes some mindset shifting, especially given that the fashion industry is trying to get you to throw away your money on cheap disposable clothing. But this process will change you, and your approach to fashion and shopping will adapt along the way. The allure of shopping fades as you find genuine joy in the clothes you already have. When you have those two-minute mornings and walk out the door in a style that is authentically you, the desire to find yourself through experimental shopping no longer has a hold on you.

One of my clients, Nancy, was a devoted bargain hunter. She rarely paid full price for anything, but she was almost always frustrated with her wardrobe. Her budget felt tight, so she assumed quality was out of reach. Once we reframed shopping as something she did *intentionally* and *infrequently*, everything shifted. Instead of chasing deals, she began saving for pieces she really loved. Buying just a few times a year allowed her to invest in clothing that fit better, lasted longer, and actually reflected her personal style. For the first time, she was excited about building her closet with perfect pieces.

Your assignment now is to open up a spreadsheet and start making your list. Make it as simple or as detailed as you want, and name it "[Name's] Master Shopping List." Enjoy filling it with items you need and want, adding information about color, styles, and prices as you go. As you add items, think about their relative importance to your overall wardrobe and Youniform needs. Finally, prioritize the top five items, then give yourself a reward for taking a big step towards changing the way you approach shopping. Even if you spend just fifteen minutes on this exercise, you'll feel more organized and clear about what actually belongs in your closet.

Holding On is Holding You Back

She sashays up the mountain, covered with snow, feeling a freedom she has never known. Emboldened and empowered, she shakes out her hair and as the musical crescendo builds, belts out *"Let it go, let it go..."* I have young daughters, so perhaps I've seen *Frozen* enough times to illustrate that scene by memory. But Elsa makes a really great point; sometimes you have to learn to let it go.

One of the biggest events of the year is our annual decluttering challenge. This is a group experience we run every January for our current and new clients. The new year brings new goals and often resolutions, and making space in your closet is a great thing to put on the agenda.

Our process is different, as we stretch it out for two full weeks so you can focus and make big progress without getting overwhelmed. For me, decluttering is a maintenance phase, but many of my clients first started with our annual decluttering challenge, only then realizing that they had plenty to learn about personal style.

I recommend all of my clients and students take this challenge, even if they've already started their Youniform journey with me, so no matter when you're reading this book, please get notified so you won't miss the next decluttering challenge. You can join my email list and pick up your bonuses at younifombook.com.

I personally love the decluttering challenge and do my best each year to participate—because even *my* closest bloats as time goes by. Even when you fully know your style, and make smart shopping decisions about ongoing purchases, the fact remains that it's never going to be perfect. You will still occasionally grab something that isn't a smart long-term choice. Then it sits in your closet, tags still attached, mocking you silently.

When you embrace decluttering as a routine for ongoing closet maintenance, you make room for getting rid of those items that don't belong. You typically also find items you put in the "maybe" category during previous decluttering sessions, that you are now ready to release.

I can't tell you how many times I ran across an item I had spent $100+ on, worn once or twice, and then ignored. The first time decluttering came up, I felt guilty about how much money I had spent, and vowed to wear it more often to prove that it was worth it. Six months later, during another decluttering session, I again had the guilty realization that I had not worn it at all in the last six months. Still stricken by the cost of the garment, I put it to the side with plans to list it on a resale site. Finally, six months later at the next decluttering session, I'm simply fed up with the item hanging in my closet and taking up space.

Hanging onto something you don't like because you spent a lot of money on it is called the Sunk-Cost Fallacy—it's the idea that we should keep something because we already paid for it. But the trouble is, by holding onto these "sunk costs," we're actually costing ourselves *more*—more time in clothes we don't feel good in, more space wasted that could hold a different garment, more emotional upset over not wearing something we "wasted" money on.

That money is gone, and I am never getting it back. *But* we can choose to let it go and stop sinking more "costs" into it. My sanity—and no longer feeling guilty about that piece of clothing—is worth more than the sad amount I will get on Poshmark, further reduced by fees and shipping. Feeling relief, I shove that item in a donation bag and move on with my life.

Yes, I have depression-era feelings and attachment to things, and clothing is one area where I have to be incredibly mindful and vicious about letting go of things. You might be like me, or maybe you have zero issues getting rid of clothing that no longer suits you. In either case, I encourage you to make regular decluttering part of your style maintenance process. Below are a few ways you can approach this task to make it work for you.

Annual Decluttering

If you choose an annual process, be aware that this is more like a project, and should be undertaken with planning and a framework. This is how we do it as a community, and we spend 14 days working through the entire closet, from tops to shoes and everything in between. Each day we ask you to try on the items in the category, and sort them into keep, donate, maybe piles. Because we are going through your entire wardrobe, this prevents burnout and also lets you focus more on areas where you have more items, or even take days off when the focus area is already under control. You can gamify these with trackers or by asking friends to do it with you.

Seasonal Decluttering

For many, this is the most logical way of approaching clothing decluttering, and it can be scheduled alongside your seasonal rotation. This works particularly well if you live in a climate with four distinct seasons. At the end of each season (we'll use winter to spring as an example), you take a simple assessment of what you have worn.

For our example, you would go through your winter wardrobe, making note of what should stay, be repaired, donated, or trashed. Then, you store those items away in a tote or separate closet out of sight. As you rotate in your spring wardrobe, you analyze each piece the same way, checking to see if it still belongs in your closet for the upcoming season. This also allows you to identify holes each season to make plans for your shopping list.

These two methods are the most useful and aligned with a curated method of approaching style through Youniforms. But there's one thing I must say you should never, ever do.

Do not ever take everything in your wardrobe out in a decluttering session. You probably have more than you realize, and this is a recipe for disaster. Some experts will tell you to take everything out of your closet and put it on the bed, going through each item and only keeping what works and discarding the rest.

But let's go back to stats. If the average woman has 150 pieces in her closet, that's a ton of clothes to manage in one sitting. If you get frustrated or tired or start struggling with self-image in the middle, you're doomed. Your two choices are either not to sleep on the bed (or hide it somewhere else), or painstakingly put it all back, which means you wasted the time. Hello more guilt. I'm gonna say *no thanks* to that.

Decluttering your clothing should be part of your process at least once a year. Your style isn't static and will demand changes, even if they are small. When you take the time to mindfully make space in your closet, it frees you up to find a newfound appreciation for the things you keep and wear and love.

Decluttering after implementing Youniforms is *much* easier.

My process now usually involves getting rid of a fifth or sixth option that I really don't love as much my 4-Piece Wardrobe items. Sometimes it's a print or color; other times, it's a slight style variation that I don't love. I usually end up decluttering shoes the most, since I prefer a slight maximalist approach and have a deep love for shoes. My clients have a similar experience over time. New clients often get rid of over 100 items, while long-term clients barely reach the fifty mark, if that. Keep in mind that includes everything from underwear to earrings. But every one of them benefits from the clarity gained by regularly cleaning out their closet.

When was the last time you took a serious look at your closet through the lens of auditing via decluttering? Whether it's been a month, a year, or never...I'd like you to take a peek right quick and look for uncut tags. These will give you a quick look at the health of your closet from this angle. No judgment here, but note down how many you find in your entire closet (shoes in boxes count too). If you have three or less, I know you've done a great job managing your closet inventory; if you have 4-10, that's what I would expect to be average. If you have more than ten, it's time to take a long hard look at your style, and choose to let some things go.

Style Is Not Meant to Stay the Same

A couple of years ago my favorite local grocery store renovated the store. It drove me absolutely bananas. I rarely go inside the grocery store (thanks to Covid-era pickups), but when I do, I have a process, and it's built based on the store layout. In this particular H-E-B, I walk past the personal care section, take the baby aisle to get to the dairy, grab my yogurt and eggs, skim the prepared breakfast meats, then weave through the aisles, finishing with chilled meat and produce. But during the renovation everything was mixed up, so running inside for a random ice cream craving meant wandering around aimlessly and angrily for a few minutes.

Your personal style is going to change.
Your body will change.
Your lifestyle will change.
Your taste and preferences will change.

Humans don't like change. I have found this to be truer with each passing year. We get set in our ways, comfortable in our routines, familiar with the status quo around us. And while some people swear change is fun (disclaimer: I kinda love it), the reality hits home when we face a disruption like the grocery store renovation.

Your personal style is going to change. Your body will change. Your lifestyle will change. Your taste and preferences will change.

This critical mental shift is something I spend a great deal of time navigating silently in the background with my clients. For many, it manifests in the desire for the "perfect" item or "perfect" closet. Even if you were to attain wardrobe perfection, it would last only for a moment, because time marches on. But once you accept and understand that your style is evolving just like you, it allows you to roll with the changes that come, instead of fighting them and staying stuck in a style rut.

Our group style program teaches all the concepts in this book, deeply and with guidance from myself and our team of experts. Each stage of the journey is mapped out with deep discovery exercises to make the process tangible and useful. Everyone is working at their own pace, each in her own stage of the journey. But every year we schedule maintenance tasks around the various parts, to help them revisit the core of their personal style and make tweaks.

As I'm writing this, I'm deciding on the topic for our monthly coaching call, and it will likely be something around color. At baseline, it will be something I've said or taught before, but I'm asking my clients to dig in, go deeper, make updates to their style. Maybe they'll reorganize their signature colors, or dive deep into how to express one of their essences for a specific Youniform type. And sometimes we push against common struggles like showing more skin in the summer confidently.

If you're looking for ongoing support, guided implementation, and a community of women walking through this process together, you can learn more about our signature style program at **iamaradiantwoman.com**.

If you are going this alone, there are several things I have outlined in this book that you should make a point of revisiting and revising at least annually. Here's a quick reminder:

1. **Update your color palette** - I typically find that color palettes get smaller as the years go by. Clients realize they don't use as many colors as they first imagined and get rid of accents. Or they planned a set of neutrals, and one is never getting worn. When you review your color palette, reorganize your closet by color, and make a note of any color holes that need filled. Add these items to your shopping list. Declutter colors you're not wearing. (See how it comes full circle?)

2. **Review your style goals** - I find these can shift a lot over the course of a year, especially from the first version to the second. As you become more in tune with your personal style, you'll see what impact you want to have, and what you want to communicate about yourself. Revisit your buckets and see if they represent who you want to be. But especially check the actual words you chose. Examine their connotations and see if they still fit, or if they are lacking. Spend some time reviewing favorite outfits to see if you were expressing yourself through your style goals or if you still have some work to do.

3. **Conduct a size and fit check** - As you've been working through the process to discover your signature style and build style Youniforms your preferences should have become more refined. You will probably have items that are okay but not great, and this is the time to review the fit of those items to see if they should stay or go. Also check your sizing to see if the clothes in your closet are still comfortable on the body you have right now. If you find holes here, be sure to add them to your shopping list.

1. **Assess the 7 Foolproof Outfits framework** - Review your existing Youniforms to see if they are meeting the needs you have in your life. Be brutally honest with yourself here. If you have two work/professional Youniforms and you recently retired, it's time to explore what other outfit types you need to focus on now. If you have a full running Youniform, but you had knee surgery ten months ago and took up swimming, review your activity Youniform to see if it meets your current needs. Allow your *current* lifestyle to dictate what gets to stay in your closet. We can only live in the present, not our past or future self.

Change is hard. And none of us are immune. But there's a way to honor those changes with a wardrobe that brings you joy, without chasing a version of you with tons of impulse buys. The Youniform Framework gives you the foundation to build a closet in modular sections, tweaking what is working, and building or discarding entire modules when they no longer fit your life.

Once you have done the hard work of finding your best colors, creating style goals, finding your essence, and honoring your body, updates to your style don't feel as hard, because the *core of you* hasn't changed. Only the outer experience. Then, style renewal becomes more like changing the curtains versus knocking down the entire wall.

How to Actually Get Dressed in Two Minutes

One of my clients recently said to me, "I love my Youniforms, and I enjoy my closet, but I still don't know how to choose what to wear each day."

I shared how I approach this every morning to make sure getting dressed is a 2-5 minute process and the astonished look on her face told me I had stumbled upon a critical teaching moment, so I decided to close this chapter with how to actually choose what to wear every day.

First, I want you to consider how you normally make this decision. For many women, the experience of getting dressed is much like described at the beginning of this book. A morning of chaos where you spend way too much time trying on several outfits before finally leaving the house in basically anything presentable.

For other women, outfit planning is a complete process, with some outlining weeks or a month in advance. For these women, the effort is spent in one big chunk, looking ahead to schedule and weather to make somewhat informed decisions. Whether you are a planner or fly-by-the-seat-of-your-pantser, the process that people use to choose their clothes can differ as well.

Outfit decisions typically fall into one of two categories: logical or emotional. The logical types look at things like weather or activities to decide what clothing is most practical for the day. The emotional types dress based on their mood, whether it's up or down, and use their clothing to moderate their mental state. Research suggests that moody dressing seems to have similar outcomes: depression means baggy clothes, feeling unattractive means defaulting to black, confidence equates to more form-fitting clothing, and good moods are bolstered by bright color choices (McKnight 2013).

But the Youniform Framework allows you to use logic and emotion when choosing your clothes, without having to default to one or the other. Because when practicality meets dopamine, amazing things happen.

For those of you thinking, *Oh, just choose your clothes the night before*, I see you too. I used to take this approach back when my closet was more chaotic. When I shared it with my community, I had several students who hated this approach. They said that their mood could change from the night before to the next morning, and they found themselves back at the starting point, completely unsure what to wear. I still recommend more intensive outfit planning for special occasions like family photos, important meetings, or speaking events. Obviously, in those moments, you want to take extra care with your appearance. But on a day-to-day basis, a modular closet of style Youniforms is a more fun and useful approach to the daily outfit struggle.

Come along with me on a typical morning decision-making process about what to wear, and see how easy it can be to go from pajamas to fully dressed in under five minutes. You open your eyes to the alarm (why are they so annoying??) and mentally prepare yourself for the day. A quick activity rundown shows you have a morning meeting, an afternoon pedicure, and a kid's baseball game in the evening. This isn't 1920, so you don't need three outfits for the day, but yours needs to cover some major ground. You realize the best choice is a dress Youniform, because you can make some tweaks to dress it up or down for the day's activities.

Now you get to play off your mood just a bit...are you in the mood for neutrals or something with a bit more color? Since you're feeling fresh and excited about the day, you choose a red subtle print dress and pair it with a navy blazer for your morning meeting. You have options for both warm and cool weather, but since it's baseball season, you choose the spring/summer options.

You know the pedicure will be better with open-toe shoes, so you grab a pair of metallic sandals to keep the professional vibe for the meeting without having to change for the afternoon. A simple necklace and dangly earrings add just the right amount of sparkle. After your meeting, you shed the blazer and keep it simple for the rest of the day. In the evening, you pull your hair up to show off the earrings, and change into casual sandals or sneakers for the ballpark.

It's the ultimate day to night dressing, but you don't have to try on five outfits to land on a winner, only to have to change midday for the casual part. But even on a less busy stay at home day, you can still use this same process to make sure you're not wearing pajamas.

You wake up leisurely without an alarm (living the life!) and realize you have nothing to do today. Some people might be content to veg out in PJs, but you know better and choose elevated loungewear. You recently splurged on some quality joggers and have a great Youniform built around them: crew neck tee and denim jacket. Because you're feeling relaxed, you decide on soothing blues: navy joggers and a light blue tee. You don't really need the jacket at home, but you grab a cozy light gray cardigan to stay warm.

As you're enjoying a nice day on the couch binge-watching Netflix, you get a text from a friend you haven't seen in three years, saying she's in town and asking to meet up for a coffee.

Since you're already dressed, this moment is an easy yes. You swap the cardigan for the jacket, throw on some basic flats and stud earrings, and out the door you go. Yes, even joggers can look intentional if you do it the right way and have a confident base that fits you well and flatters in your best colors. You get to enjoy the surprise visit with an old friend and a warm cup of coffee, feeling comfy and cozy, but still fully dressed. There was no panic, which is what a great wardrobe does for any day.

The power of Youniform dressing is that you always have the right clothes to wear, from big meetings to lazy Saturdays to the morning drop-off line at school. Each day you look completely put together. Every day you show up as *your* version of the stylish woman, because you have grown into her.

From the way you shop mindfully, to your regular ruthless decluttering process, and your commitment to making small shifts to your style to reflect the person you are becoming, you embody what it means to be truly stylish.

You no longer worry about what other people think about your clothes, because you love them. Your mornings are easy, and getting dressed is now fun and creative, instead of stressful and overwhelming.

Chapter Ten Highlights

- A truly stylish wardrobe functions as a management system, not a static collection of clothes.
- Once your Youniforms are established, shopping should shift from browsing to filling clearly defined gaps.
- A master shopping list replaces impulse buying with priority-based, intentional wardrobe growth.
- Limiting purchases to a ranked top five items keeps your closet cohesive while allowing flexibility and joy.
- Regular decluttering is a maintenance practice that protects clarity, reduces decision fatigue, and prevents sunk-cost guilt.
- Personal style must be revisited and adjusted as body, lifestyle, and preferences change over time.
- Daily outfit decisions become effortless when logic (needs) and emotion (mood) are both supported by modular Youniforms.

Eleven

Get Dressed. Be Radiant.

"No legacy is so rich as honesty." - William Shakespeare

By the time you've reached this final chapter, you've already done the hardest part. You've stopped treating style like a guessing game and started approaching it with intention. You understand why getting dressed used to feel so frustrating, and you've built a system that makes choosing clothes simple, repeatable, and aligned with your real life. Now, it's time to talk about what that simplicity makes possible.

In the beginning I promised you this wasn't a book about fashion, and even though we talked about the industry, this process isn't really about how to be more stylish, or trendy, or buy the latest thing to look cool. It's about these two simple acts:

Get dressed, quickly, efficiently, in clothes you love to wear, that are flattering by design, and work for the life you're living right now. So that you can *be radiant* every moment of the day. With every interaction with your most important people, you create a lasting memory, and make a positive change in the world.

I started this journey because I was miserable in my clothes and I craved simplicity and fun in my closet. The mix of capsule wardrobe and cozy dresses became my message and driving force. When I started, I never expected to end up here. But I can see the future of myself, this beautiful business, and a multitude of women experiencing freedom and confidence with a Youniform closet.

The Youniform Framework was an aha moment, a realization of something I had been exposed to my whole life, and done intuitively before giving it a fancy title. From wearing a school uniform in first grade to creating a framework, I was made for this message. But along the way, I unlocked confidence and more that I had been missing.

I have laughed and cried with my clients. I have watched them have moments of intense realization that they are worthy and beautiful.

I spent my teens struggling to fit in, my twenties going absolutely wild, unlocking my dreams only to find faith, and my thirties experiencing the transformative joy of becoming a mom. And even though my old self died in the process, I've never missed a moment of my previous life. I didn't care that I was still wearing maternity clothes when my baby was actually a toddler. No one noticed if I wore my hair in a messy mom bun six days out of seven (or just cut it off for ease). My little kids under five didn't notice if I weighed an extra forty pounds.

I didn't expect to be a successful personal stylist. I probably would have laughed at you if you had suggested decades ago this would be my "thing." But as an old friend said to me when I told her, "Oh, that makes sense for you, actually." So I guess my love for pretty things and clothes has been a constant my whole life. My younger self would have considered it vain, and my current self sometimes thinks it's somewhat shallow.

But then I see what it unlocks, and I realize I'm wrong (both then and now).

One of my clients reaches out and tells me a story about how amazing she feels, and how her husband actually noticed her and gave her a compliment, and how she went to an event and walked in gracefully and confidently. Another posts a win in our style community, sharing how she went shopping and bought nothing on impulse because she loved her Youniform closet better. And a member who has been silent for months comes back ready to keep exploring her style and finding herself in a new season.

My desire for simplicity has opened doors for me to see real transformation in other women, and that is a gift I never expected.

I have laughed and cried with my clients. I have watched them have moments of intense realization that they are worthy and beautiful.

It is a privilege, and all of it exists because, one day, I was so frustrated getting dressed that I decided to do something about it. Professionally, this means I get to build bigger, dream harder, think about how I can expand the influence of this message.

Personally, it has changed my life. It has helped support the logistics of raising a large family in a shaky economy. My closet is what I always dreamed of, filled with clothes I love to wear. Every day I get to dress on the whim of which of my favorite things I feel like putting on, colorful prints or beautiful rich solids. I can admire and appreciate every style and color that comes out, while confidently knowing that only a small few are actually for me. My relationships are richer because I grew as a person, holding boundaries and standing firm in who I am.

Style exploration is personal exploration, and as you find yourself, you get stronger.

It's hard for me to bring this book to an end, because the truth is, there's no finish line to what creating a Youniform means to you and your life. Every day it gives back to you — time, joy, and confidence. We are changing constantly, and our closets and style need to evolve with us, helping us express timeless beauty.

But there is one more thing I absolutely must say about this journey:

The Youniform is not the destination.

It is a system that supports becoming a Radiant Woman, so that you are free to live a Radiant Life.

Your Morning Sets the Tone for Your Whole Day

A Radiant Life means that your days are filled with things that matter, and you seek to minimize things that don't. One of those things is the time you spend getting dressed, because you want to show up for the people you love and give them your best. Spending over five minutes making that decision is no longer acceptable, because you're not willing to steal it from them.

Instead, your personal style now creates a rhythm in your life, anchored by those easy mornings getting dressed in one of your Youniforms, and going on with your day confidently.

Your closet is a showcase of beauty, organized cohesively into your categories, and a few color families steal the show, with occasional pops of accent colors. In the cooler months, your colors shift deeper and richer, but everything is cohesive and beautiful. But even more important, you are no longer drawn to colors that don't work for you (just because they're trending). You acknowledge them in passing and continue wearing what makes you glow.

And when those trends veer into a different cut of jeans, or some version of blazers that you know looks bad on you, you never consider buying them "just because." Now you have the self-assurance to enjoy looking at them on other people—the ladies who look stunning in those styles—and know that beauty comes in many forms, and acknowledge there is something unique for everyone.

Looking in the mirror no longer stresses you out. Sure, maybe there are some extra lines and gray hair (how lucky are we to gain wisdom with age?) and a few stubborn pounds. But the woman in the mirror has a purpose and meaning, and the clothing you wear is simply a reflection of your heart. You walk past it most of the time like any other piece of furniture, on your way to call a friend, or get that promotion you've worked hard to earn.

Regardless of what the day holds, you no longer approach getting dressed without a plan. You know exactly what you have to wear because your closet is organized around repeatable Youniforms that support your real life. Work, community casual, casual at home, hobbies, events—each context already has options waiting for you.

Some days that means wearing your work Youniform. Other days it's a casual-at-home Youniform, or one of your dress-based combinations that can flex across multiple settings. You don't need a dozen different silhouettes anymore, and you don't rely on luck to feel put together.

This is what it looks like when getting dressed becomes your zone of genius. People notice. Compliments come easily. Others assume you have a secret; but the truth is simpler than that. You stopped dressing mindlessly and started dressing with intention. You understand now that no one else can design your closet for you, because no one else lives your life.

When you simplify your closet with personal Youniforms, you automatically think less about yourself.

When you sit down at your computer to check your email, you don't get sucked into online window shopping and *add to cart* old habits. You get excited for your planned shopping seasons, and you get to buy quality garments that fill existing gaps in your closet, and maybe even splurge on a great pair of shoes or Italian leather handbag.

And once a year, you approach any excess with brutal precision, carving away at things that no longer work for the life you have *this year.* Flattering colors you never wore, prints you didn't love, a pair of shoes you never chose. You're able to let go with no lingering guilt or emotions, because you know your Youniform closet functions like a perfect machine, helping you to embody the woman you have become *for this time.*

You recognize that your style is an ongoing process, and the stages in the background of the Youniform Framework keep you moving. Just as you evolve every year into a more beautiful butterfly, your closet keeps moving with you. Getting dressed is fun and exciting and you get compliments, but even more, it's a routine act, as simple as brushing your teeth, but as profound as leaving a legacy.

Make Great Style Part of Your Legacy

Remember the game M.A.S.H. you played as a kid with your friends? Mansion, apartment, shack, house...none of us ever wanted to end up with the shack. Whether you played a short version, or you created the longest future quiz ever, you were dreaming about the future. I want to be a doctor when I grow up, or I'm going to marry Brad (thank goodness, I didn't!). Wishing and dreaming of a big life was easy when the whole thing stretched ahead of you.

But what about now? What does dreaming look like these days?

It's hard to think of something brighter in the future when you're struggling in the day-to-day. I have had clients over the years who couldn't get out of the daily overwhelm. Some of them I still follow, and I see their lives are much the same as they were when I met them. Because purpose and legacy require forward motion, and they didn't decide to get into motion. You have to take the first step, and do one simple action, for anything to change.

And the reason we dream is because we desire change. We know deep down that we are created for a greater purpose.

Whether that's family, or community, or even changing the world, we each have a mission to fulfill. And every great mission revolves around enriching the lives of other people. The second greatest commandment in the Bible is to love others as yourself. It's a given that we love ourselves: that we instinctively focus on actions that make ourselves look better and meet our needs. But if we get trapped here, we miss out on accomplishing our life's work.

Then there is no legacy, no lasting meaning, no heartfelt eulogies at our funeral. We are forgotten because we failed to create anything of value. And the reason we failed to be memorable is that we were too focused on ourselves.

When you simplify your closet with personal Youniforms, you automatically think less about yourself.

Instead, you get to quickly get dressed, and go forth into meaningful work: reading books to your kids, encouraging a friend over coffee, leading a meeting with passion, investing in a new venture with confidence, making decisions that will echo for generations.

This is what sets the Youniform Framework apart from every other approach to style. It doesn't tell you who you should be. Instead, it quietly removes the constant focus on yourself by giving you a system that works.

Getting dressed becomes both efficient and enjoyable, without sacrificing expression, and without requiring daily effort or second-guessing.

Most style systems are visually inspiring but not truly functional for real life. They aren't built to account for the nuances of different seasons, responsibilities, or callings. The Youniform Framework is.

It's designed for you to embrace your individuality with efficiency, so your energy goes toward your legacy, instead of being consumed by what you're wearing.

With all of this in mind, write one powerful statement beginning with, "I want to be remembered as someone who..."

When you consider this statement, view it through the long lens of personal style and imagine what that person looks like. If it's hard to imagine, or the vision is blurry, congratulations, you have discovered the truth: no one will remember what you wear.

But everyone will remember who you really were.

Your clothing is the pathway to the life you were meant to lead. It is a tool that you wield every day to create action and meaning.

Never lose sight of your dreams and legacy, but let them lead you into the best version of yourself today.

Becoming a Radiant Woman

Many years ago, I began a program for women to walk hand in hand through this journey of personal style. I called it the Radiant Woman Intensive (and it was super intense because, spoiler; I don't know how to do shallow). It has been renamed, but the Radiant Woman part remains.

Earlier this year, I considered changing it to something more system-sounding, to reflect the changes here in this book. Then, in a moment of divine will, I dealt with a trademark infringement. In the process of defending the mark—and the soul-searching I did in the dark moments—I remembered how pivotal this phrase is to the transformation my clients get.

It's never just clothes.

It's always a turning-inside-out, tearing down thoughts that have been broken for too long, and filling those gaps with confidence, beauty, and a life that is intensely focused on meaning.

I am a Radiant Woman.

These are the words my clients repeat when they come full circle in this process of style resurrection. I have been privileged to serve hundreds of women, and if I polled them, I could likely find dozens of stories of moments where life shifts dramatically, and their simplified Youniform closet made life easier. But here are a few I am more intimately familiar with:

Jeanine drifted into my life by design. She's a business coach who mentored me in exchange for style advice. In the first year I met her, she burned her original business down and pivoted to a new process. She had hired stylists before that had come and built her the perfect wardrobe to the tune of thousands. But she still felt unhappy and unsettled with her closet. As her business pivot took off, she began waking up at 4 am to write a book about her process. She told me that clearing the mental clutter around what to wear made a big dent in her ability to hold that space daily for months. She created a blue ocean in her area of expertise and now has several books, expanding her business and her place in the industry.

Lily is one of my very first color analysis clients right from the beginning. She loyally jumps into every new program I offer, committed to seeking and finding her internal self. She had some deep wounds from devastating trials as a mom, and those have affected how she saw herself, including her self-worth. As she grew more confident in herself, she gained the courage to leave an abusive marriage. Her confidence and contentment have never been higher, and I love to see the peace she has now in who she is.

Hannah is a new client, and somewhat quiet in her style journey. She enjoys experimenting and examining herself intentionally and introspectively. Last year she all but disappeared, but it was to move cross-country over a staged period of several months. Periodically she would pop in and share how it was going living out of a suitcase, and express gratitude that she had a solid grasp on her personal style, and could be joyful with her Youniforms while living minimalist.

What will the simplicity of Youniforms do for you?

On the day my son needed stitches, I wasn't dressed. My oldest boy at the time was four and climbing up the back of the La-Z-Boy recliner when he tumbled off and hit his chin on the windowsill on the way to the floor. He stood up screaming, blood running down his face, and my heart jumped. I stopped the bleeding and looked at the gaping cut space under his chin. I was still in my pajamas, hair crazy and completely unprepared for a surprise trip to urgent care. Back then I probably did what most people do: threw on the quickest clean item I could find, hid my hair, and rushed out the door, maybe remembering to put on deodorant. That moment reflected my state of being: messy mom life.

But through this book, you have learned that your style should be the gateway to a bigger life. Just like messy mom was only for that stage, getting control of my closet and finding my personal style has made me a put-together (still a little messy) mom. I spent years searching for the perfect closet, only to realize that the Youniforms I had been wearing for decades were the only answer I needed.

I hope this book has opened your eyes to the power of simplified dressing. I have shared with you the process of creating repeatable outfits for every part of your life, and how to find the perfect style to express yourself. Take a moment to reflect on all that you have learned and consider these questions:

1. What is the biggest insight you have gained from this book?

2. What's your first priority for changing your wardrobe?

3. Write down your biggest remaining question or challenge and email it to us at admin@radiantlydressed.com. We read them all!

Your style is always communicating something, whether or not you mean to. Let's be sure you're saying what you want to say.

If you would like help walking this journey, I would love to invite you to join our premium style coaching program for women. Inside this exclusive program, you'll work through these answers with guidance from your personal stylist and support from a community of women who are simplifying their closets so they can amplify their calling. If you're ready to stop letting your closet steal time from the best things in your life, I'd love to welcome you inside.

You were created to live a life of purpose, to be a light and beacon to those around you. There is freedom in exactly that version of yourself, even if you don't know her yet. Don't let frazzled mornings getting dressed steal from you the legacy that is meant to be yours.

Get Dressed. Be Radiant.

Chapter Eleven Highlights

- Getting dressed is not the point; freeing your time, energy, and attention for what matters most is.
- The Youniform is not about self-expression alone, but about removing daily friction so you can live with clarity and purpose.
- When your closet works on repeat, you naturally stop thinking about yourself and start showing up more fully for others.
- Style becomes powerful when it supports your life quietly, instead of demanding constant effort, decision-making, or validation.
- A Radiant Woman is not remembered for what she wore, but for the life she lived once getting dressed stopped getting in the way.

Appendix A: ColorEssence Seasons

In chapters seven and eight I shared with you the concepts of color analysis and essence. While I was writing this book, I was also developing a proprietary color analysis system with my clients that bridges both of these style theories. Currently, I offer this in our Comprehensive Style Report, and will be expanding this system into digital and physical products. Perhaps it will even be my next book!

In an effort to help you integrate these two powerful concepts, I present to you the ColorEssence Seasons.

System Overview

The ColorEssence System is a refined approach to personal style that integrates the Big Four Seasons with the seven style essences, creating a seamless way to understand both one's best colors and the most natural way to express them through style. This system is designed to balance color harmony with essence-driven styling, ensuring that every woman can enhance her unique beauty with confidence and ease.

Each person is typed using three key identifiers:

- Big Four Color Season – One of the four traditional seasonal palettes: Winter, Spring, Summer, or Autumn
- Essence Type – One of four descriptive categories based on style essences:
    - Flowy (Natural & Ethereal)
    - Bold (Dramatic & Romantic)
    - Playful (Gamine & Ingenue)
    - Classic (Classic)
- Energy Balance – A designation of T (Soft/Yin) or G (Strong/Yang) to reflect whether the dominant essence leans toward a gentler or stronger expression of the season.

This results in sixteen total style profiles, each combining season, essence type, and energy balance to create a cohesive and individualized style identity.

The Four Essence Types & Their Styling Influence

- Flowy types bring an organic, effortless feel to their season. Their style prioritizes soft draping, movement, and an unstructured aesthetic, creating a sense of ethereal or natural ease.

- Bold types create a high-impact, striking look within their season. Whether through rich colors, dramatic styling, or luxurious elements, they command attention and exude presence.
- Playful types add a youthful, light, and animated energy to their season. Their style thrives on small-scale details, crisp tailoring, and lively color combinations, giving a fresh, vibrant aesthetic.
- Classic types reflect balance, elegance, and refinement within their season. Their style is timeless, symmetrical, and polished, creating a sophisticated, harmonious presence.

Soft (T) vs. Strong (G) Energy Balance

Each essence type can be further refined by the T or G designation:

- T (Soft/Yin): A gentler approach to the essence, with a more blended, graceful, or romantic feel. These individuals often prefer smooth transitions, softer textures, and an understated elegance.
- G (Strong/Yang): A more defined, structured, or high-contrast expression of the essence. These individuals can handle sharper contrasts, bolder styling choices, and more pronounced details.

ColorEssence Spring Seasons

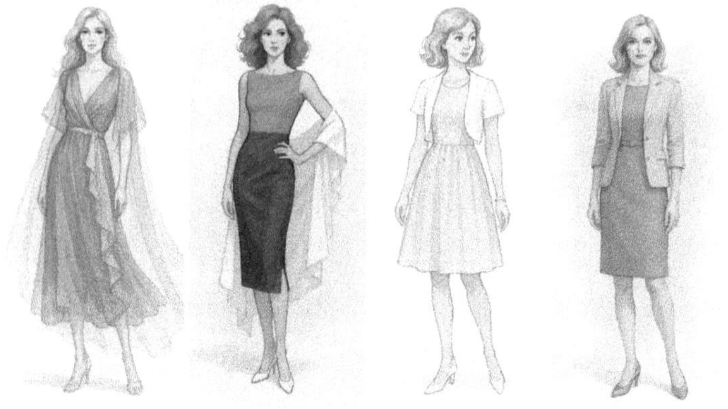

Figure A1 Illustrations of ColorEssence Spring Types

Flowy Spring

The *Flowy Spring* type combines the warm, bright coloring of Spring with the fluid, unstructured nature of the Natural and/or Ethereal style essences. While Spring's palette is typically clear and energetic, the influence of these essences softens its vibrancy, creating a more effortless and organic feel.

Sunlit, fresh, and watercolor-like hues remain flattering, but they are best expressed through flowing silhouettes, soft draping, and lightweight or textured fabrics that enhance movement. Instead of structured tailoring or crisp contrast, the Flowy Spring thrives in delicate layering, airy shapes, and an overall sense of lightness, blending Spring's natural warmth and luminosity with an unforced, graceful elegance.

The G designation indicates an undercurrent of strong, yang energy within this blend. This adds a sense of presence and quiet

intensity to the otherwise soft and free-flowing style, creating a balance between movement and definition. A Flowy Spring G can carry richer or more dynamic shades from the Spring palette with ease, and their style benefits from an intentional approach—flowing, but with a sense of structure that keeps it from feeling too relaxed.

The T designation indicates a softer, more yin energy within this blend. This brings an overall gentleness to the light and fresh tones of Spring, allowing for a more seamless and blended approach to color. A Flowy Spring T may gravitate toward the softer or more pastel shades within the Spring palette, favoring delicate transitions over bold contrasts. Their style is best expressed through light, sheer layers, soft movement, and fabrics that create a dreamy, weightless effect without overwhelming their natural fluidity.

Bold Spring

The *Bold Spring* type combines the warm, bright coloring of Spring with the intense, striking nature of the Dramatic and/or Romantic style essences. While Spring's palette is typically fresh and energetic, the influence of these essences amplifies its vibrancy, creating a look that is high-impact, confident, and full of presence.

Golden corals, vivid turquoise, bright greens, and crisp yellows remain flattering, but they are best expressed through bold styling choices, eye-catching color combinations, and statement details that emphasize movement and energy. Instead of soft blending or subtle transitions, the Bold Spring thrives in high-saturation hues, luxurious textures, and an overall sense of dynamic glamour, whether through striking contrasts or radiant, high-energy styling.

The G designation indicates an undercurrent of strong, yang energy within this blend. This adds a commanding, high-energy presence, reinforcing Spring's natural brightness with sharp contrasts and structured styling. A Bold Spring G can easily wear the most intense, saturated colors from the palette and benefits from styling that leans into strong, confident shapes, bold accessories, and a vibrant, lively aesthetic.

The T designation indicates a softer, more yin energy within this blend. This enhances the alluring, luminous side of the Spring palette, creating a look that is bold yet fluid and enchanting. A Bold Spring T may favor plush, flowing fabrics, soft drapes, and radiant details that maintain intensity while preserving a sense of charm and warmth.

Playful Spring

The *Playful Spring* type combines the warm, bright coloring of Spring with the youthful, small-scale nature of the Gamine and/or Ingenue style essences. While Spring's palette is naturally energetic and fresh, the influence of these essences enhances its light, lively, and whimsical quality, creating a look that is cheerful, charming, and full of movement.

Warm pastels, vivid citrus tones, and clear, fresh brights remain flattering, but they are best expressed through small-scale patterns, tailored yet animated silhouettes, and fun, eye-catching details that enhance their natural effervescence. Instead of long, flowing lines or heavy structure, the Playful Spring thrives in bouncy shapes, crisp detailing, and an overall sense of joyful vibrancy, blending Spring's lively radiance with an energetic, youthful essence.

The G designation indicates an undercurrent of strong, yang energy within this blend. This adds a punchy, bold playfulness to the Playful Spring aesthetic, reinforcing sharp contrasts, high-energy styling, and structured yet vibrant outfits. A Playful Spring G naturally carries saturated brights, color blocking, and tailored but animated pieces, benefiting from snappy details, quirky accessories, and an expressive, dynamic presence.

The T designation indicates a softer, more yin energy within this blend. This enhances the sweet, delicate side of the Spring palette, creating a look that is playful yet soft and enchanting. A Playful Spring T may gravitate toward lighter pastels, rounded shapes, and soft textures, favoring gentle ruffles, dainty prints, and an overall sense of warmth and charm that maintains Spring's brightness in a more delicate way.

Classic Spring

The *Classic Spring* type combines the warm, bright coloring of Spring with the timeless, refined nature of the Classic essence. While Spring's palette is naturally energetic and radiant, the influence of Classic brings a sense of order, symmetry, and polish, resulting in a look that is cheerful yet composed, vibrant yet sophisticated.

Clear brights, warm neutrals, and soft, sunlit pastels remain flattering, but they are best expressed through tailored silhouettes, smooth textures, and classic styling that enhances balance and elegance. Instead of overly playful shapes or dramatic contrast, the Classic Spring thrives in refined color combinations, structured layering, and an overall sense of polished vitality—blending Spring's freshness with Classic harmony and poise.

The G designation indicates an undercurrent of strong, yang energy within this blend. This adds a commanding crispness and focus to the Classic Spring aesthetic, reinforcing clean lines, sharp details, and a confident presence. A Classic Spring G wears the most vibrant, well-defined colors of the palette with clarity and benefits from sleek tailoring, bold-but-refined accessories, and an energetic yet poised silhouette.

The T designation indicates a softer, more yin energy within this blend. This enhances the sweet, graceful quality of the Spring palette, creating a look that is classic yet warm and inviting. A Classic Spring T may gravitate toward the lighter end of the palette, favoring softly structured pieces, smooth finishes, and delicate color pairings that maintain brightness without overwhelming their natural lightness. Their style is best expressed through timeless shapes, gentle contrasts, and an elegant, sunlit charm.

ColorEssence Summer Seasons

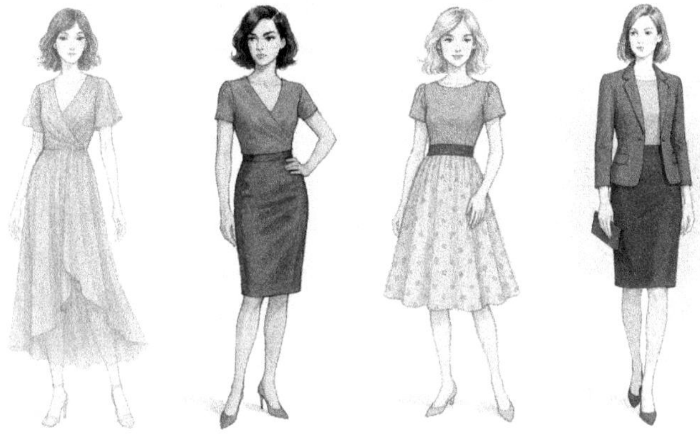

Figure A2 Illustrations representing ColorEssence Summer Types

Flowy Summer

The *Flowy Summer* type combines the cool, muted coloring of Summer with the fluid, unstructured nature of the Natural and/or Ethereal style essences. While Summer's palette is typically soft and blended, the influence of these essences enhances its gentle, flowing nature, creating a look that feels effortlessly graceful and organic.

Misty pastels, soft watercolors, and muted jewel tones remain flattering, but they are best expressed through draping silhouettes, airy layers, and delicate textures that enhance movement. Instead of sharp contrast or tailored structure, the Flowy Summer thrives in soft transitions, cascading shapes, and an overall sense of fluid refinement, blending Summer's elegant coolness with an ethereal, effortless flow.

The G designation indicates an undercurrent of strong, yang energy within this blend. This adds a quiet strength and a sense of presence to the otherwise soft and weightless aesthetic. A Flowy Summer G can carry richer or more dramatic muted tones from the Summer palette with ease, and their style benefits from long, flowing lines with an intentional structure, preventing the look from becoming too delicate or ungrounded.

The T designation indicates a softer, more yin energy within this blend. This brings an even greater sense of lightness and harmony to the naturally soft Summer palette, allowing for a seamless, dreamy quality. A Flowy Summer T may gravitate toward the most delicate and misty hues within the Summer range, favoring soft, diffused colors over defined contrasts. Their style is best expressed through feather-light layers, sheer fabrics, and gentle, organic draping that enhance their natural sense of elegance.

Bold Summer

The *Bold Summer* type combines the cool, muted coloring of Summer with the intense, striking nature of the Dramatic and/or Romantic style essences. While Summer's palette is typically soft and blended, the influence of these essences heightens its impact, creating a look that is sophisticated, high-energy, and undeniably noticeable.

Dusky roses, deep sapphires, soft plums, and misty teals remain flattering, but they are best expressed through bold styling choices, rich textures, and statement details that bring presence to Summer's otherwise delicate hues. Instead of fading into soft transitions or subtle blends, the Bold Summer thrives in intentional color contrasts, sumptuous fabrics, and an overall sense of elegant drama, whether through high-impact styling or an air of refined glamour.

The G designation indicates an undercurrent of strong, yang energy within this blend. This adds an edge of presence and intensity, reinforcing Summer's cool elegance with a sharper, more striking contrast. A Bold Summer G naturally carries the deeper and more pigmented shades of the palette and benefits from styling that leans into bold accessories, sleek finishes, and an air of quiet confidence.

The T designation indicates a softer, more yin energy within this blend. This enhances the romantic, luxurious side of the Summer palette, creating a look that is bold yet graceful and inviting. A Bold Summer T may favor plush, fluid fabrics, soft embellishments, and layered details that maintain visual impact while preserving a sense of elegance and ease.

Playful Summer

The *Playful Summer* type combines the cool, muted coloring of Summer with the youthful, small-scale nature of the Gamine and/or Ingenue style essences. While Summer's palette is typically soft and elegant, the influence of these essences infuses it with a sense of lightness, charm, and animated energy, creating a look that is delicate, lively, and effortlessly graceful.

Dusty pastels, soft watercolors, and cool floral tones remain flattering, but they are best expressed through smaller-scale patterns, tailored yet airy silhouettes, and refined yet playful details that enhance their natural lightness. Instead of long, sweeping lines or heavy contrasts, the Playful Summer thrives in soft yet structured shapes, delicate prints, and an overall sense of gentle vibrancy, blending Summer's cool sophistication with an expressive, youthful essence.

The G designation indicates an undercurrent of strong, yang energy within this blend. This adds a crisp, refined energy to the Playful Summer aesthetic, reinforcing sharper details and clean yet light contrast. A Playful Summer G naturally carries the deeper or more defined colors of the Summer palette and benefits from snappy tailoring, polishedaccessories, and an elegant but spirited presence.

The T designation indicates a softer, more yin energy within this blend. This enhances the sweet, dreamy side of the Summer palette, creating a look that is playful yet soft and romantic. A Playful Summer T may gravitate toward the lightest and airiest Summer hues, rounded shapes, and delicate fabrics, favoring gentle ruffles, flowing details, and a soft, enchanting charm that maintains Summer's grace in a more whimsical way.

Classic Summer

The *Classic Summer* type combines the cool, muted coloring of Summer with the timeless, balanced nature of the Classic essence. While Summer's palette is naturally soft and blended, the influence of Classic refines its gentle tones into a polished, harmonious aesthetic, creating a look that is elegant, structured, and effortlessly sophisticated.

Soft pastels, cool neutrals, and dusky jewel tones remain flattering, but they are best expressed through clean lines, tailored silhouettes, and high-quality fabrics that enhance balance and refinement. Instead of exaggerated softness or overly casual styles, the Classic Summer thrives in understated luxury, fluid but structured fits, and an overall sense of timeless grace, blending Summer's natural softness with a poised, traditional essence.

The G designation indicates an undercurrent of strong, yang energy within this blend. This adds a sense of presence and quiet

authority to the Classic Summer aesthetic, reinforcing structured tailoring, crisp detailing, and a polished, confident look. A Classic Summer G naturally carries the deeper and more defined shades of the Summer palette and benefits from sleek, minimal styling, fine fabrics, and refined accessories that exude effortless composure.

The T designation indicates a softer, more yin energy within this blend. This enhances the gentle, graceful side of the Summer palette, creating a look that is classic yet delicate and inviting. A Classic Summer T may gravitate toward softer pastels, lightweight but structured fabrics, and smooth textures, favoring elegant draping and timeless simplicity that maintains Summer's cool refinement with a more approachable charm.

ColorEssence Autumn Seasons

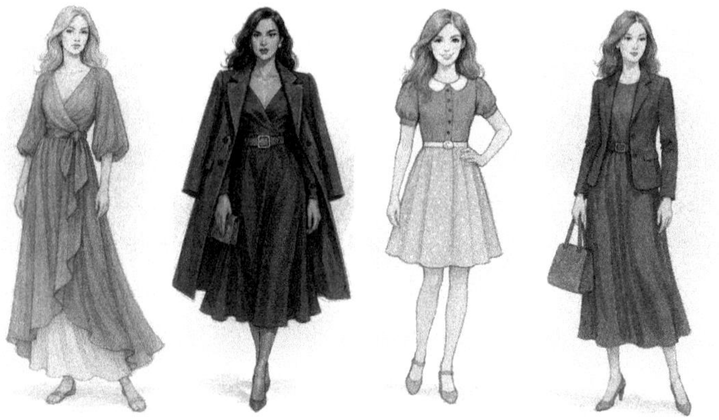

Figure A3 Illustrations representing ColorEssence Autumn Types

Flowy Autumn

The *Flowy Autumn* type combines the warm, rich coloring of Autumn with the fluid, unstructured nature of the Natural and/or Ethereal style essences. While Autumn's palette is typically deep and earthy, the influence of these essences softens its density, creating a look that feels more organic, flowing, and effortless.

Golden hues, rich browns, and deep, warm jewel tones remain flattering, but they are best expressed through draping silhouettes, soft layering, and textured fabrics that create movement and depth. Instead of structured tailoring or heavy fabrics, the Flowy Autumn thrives in organic shapes, cascading lines, and an overall sense of relaxed refinement, blending the richness of Autumn with an airy, effortless grace.

The G designation indicates an undercurrent of strong, yang energy within this blend. This adds a sense of presence and grounded intensity to the otherwise fluid and unstructured aesthetic. A Flowy Autumn G can carry deeper, more intense shades from the Autumn palette with ease, and their style benefits from flowing garments with an intentional shape, ensuring the look remains rooted and defined rather than overly loose.

The T designation indicates a softer, more yin energy within this blend. This brings a gentle, harmonious quality to the naturally rich and warm Autumn palette, allowing for a more blended and subtle approach to contrast. A Flowy Autumn T may gravitate toward the lighter, more muted earth tones, favoring soft, organic transitions over bold distinctions. Their style is best expressed through fluid draping, warm layers, and fabrics with an airy yet natural feel that enhance their effortless elegance.

Bold Autumn

The *Bold Autumn* type combines the warm, rich coloring of Autumn with the intense, striking nature of the Dramatic and/or Romantic style essences. While Autumn's palette is naturally deep and grounded, the influence of these essences amplifies its impact, creating a look that is powerful, opulent, and undeniably bold.

Golden ambers, deep rusts, rich teals, and intense earthy hues remain flattering, but they are best expressed through high-impact styling, luxurious textures, and statement details that exude confidence. Instead of soft blending or understated tones, the Bold Autumn thrives in bold color pairings, sumptuous fabrics, and an overall sense of depth and richness, whether through dramatic contrasts or glamorous, high-energy elements.

The G designation indicates an undercurrent of strong, yang energy within this blend. This adds a sense of dominance and strength, reinforcing Autumn's naturally rich and grounded aesthetic. A Bold Autumn G can carry the deepest, most intense hues of the season with ease and benefits from styling that leans into strong contrasts, bold accessories, and a commanding presence.

The T designation indicates a softer, more yin energy within this blend. This enhances the sensual, luxurious side of the Autumn palette, creating a look that is bold yet warm and inviting. A Bold Autumn T may favor plush, draped fabrics, rich details, and elegant layering that maintains intensity without relying on harsh structure, allowing for a powerful yet alluring and captivating presence.

Playful Autumn

The *Playful Autumn* type combines the warm, rich coloring of Autumn with the youthful, small-scale nature of the Gamine and/or Ingenue style essences. While Autumn's palette is typically deep and grounded, the influence of these essences infuses it with lightness, energy, and a touch of whimsy, creating a look that is warm, lively, and delightfully charming.

Golden ambers, soft cinnamons, warm olives, and rich teals remain flattering, but they are best expressed through small-scale patterns, structured yet playful silhouettes, and unique, eye-catching details that add freshness and movement. Instead of long flowing lines or deep, dramatic contrasts, the Playful Autumn thrives in layered textures, animated shapes, and an overall sense of warmth and vibrancy, blending Autumn's earthy richness with an expressive, youthful essence.

The G designation indicates an undercurrent of strong, yang energy within this blend. This adds a punchy, dynamic quality to the Playful Autumn aesthetic, reinforcing bold details and confident styling choices. A Playful Autumn G naturally carries the more vibrant, high-energy tones of the Autumn palette and benefits from snappy tailoring, structured layers, and expressive accessories that enhance their energetic, charismatic presence.

The T designation indicates a softer, more yin energy within this blend. This enhances the sweet, delicate side of the Autumn palette, creating a look that is playful yet soft and inviting. A Playful Autumn T may gravitate toward lighter, golden hues, rounded details, and soft textures, favoring gentle patterns, cozy layers, and a warm, whimsical charm that maintains Autumn's richness in a more delicate, lighthearted way.

Classic Autumn

The *Classic Autumn* type combines the warm, rich coloring of Autumn with the timeless, refined nature of the Classic essence. While Autumn's palette is known for its earthy depth and natural richness, the influence of Classic brings structure, balance, and an air of sophistication, resulting in a look that is elegant, grounded, and enduring.

Deep olives, golden browns, warm burgundies, and rich greens remain flattering, but they are best expressed through clean lines, harmonious color pairings, and polished, high-quality fabrics. Instead of casual draping or intense contrasts, the Classic Autumn thrives in tailored silhouettes, smooth textures, and an overall sense of composed, traditional beauty—blending Autumn's warmth with Classic symmetry and precision.

The G designation indicates an undercurrent of strong, yang energy within this blend. This adds strength and structure to the Classic Autumn aesthetic, reinforcing sharp tailoring, defined lines, and a sense of confident poise. A Classic Autumn G wears the deeper, more saturated tones of Autumn with grace and benefits from streamlined outfits, structured accessories, and a commanding, composed presence.

The T designation indicates a softer, more yin energy within this blend. This softens the edges of the Classic Autumn look, creating an elegant yet approachable charm. A Classic Autumn T may favor smoother blends of color, gently tailored pieces, and softly refined details that maintain structure while offering comfort and warmth. Their style radiates grace, balance, and a quiet, timeless sophistication.

ColorEssence Winter Seasons

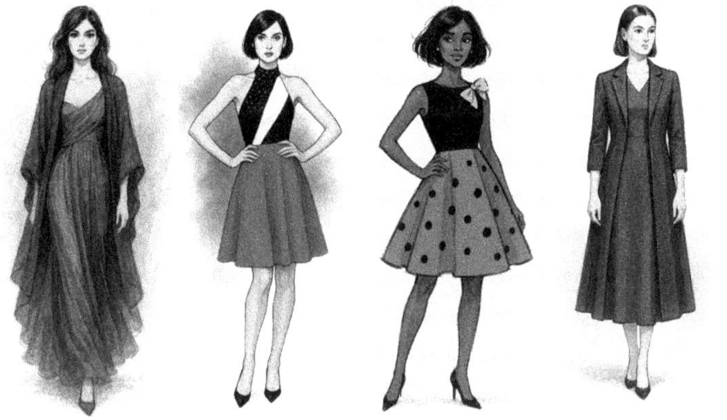

Figure A4 Illustrations representing ColorEssence Winter Types

Flowy Winter

The *Flowy Winter* type combines the cool, high-contrast coloring of Winter with the fluid, unstructured nature of the Natural and/or Ethereal style essences. While Winter's palette is typically bold and intense, the influence of these essences softens its sharp edges, creating a more effortless and organic feel.

Deep, icy, and jewel-toned hues remain flattering, but they are best expressed through flowing silhouettes, soft draping, and lightweight or textured fabrics that enhance movement. Instead of rigid tailoring or stark contrasts, the Flowy Winter thrives in elegant layering, elongated shapes, and an overall sense of refined ease, blending the striking depth of Winter with an airy, unforced grace.

The G designation indicates an undercurrent of strong, yang energy within this blend. This adds a sense of presence and quiet

intensity to the otherwise fluid and unstructured style, creating a balance between softness and strength. A Flowy Winter G can carry deeper, more dramatic shades from the Winter palette with ease, and their style benefits from a sense of deliberate movement rather than excessive looseness.

The T designation indicates a softer, more yin energy within this blend. This brings an overall gentleness to the cool, striking tones of Winter, allowing for a more subtle and blended approach to contrast. A Flowy Winter T may gravitate toward the lighter or more muted end of the Winter palette, favoring smoky or diffused colors over stark, high-contrast combinations. Their style is best expressed through delicate draping, soft layering, and fabrics with a gentle, flowing quality that enhances their natural elegance without feeling overpowering.

Bold Winter

The *Bold Winter* type combines the cool, high-contrast coloring of Winter with the intense, striking nature of the Dramatic and/or Romantic style essences. While Winter's palette is already vivid and commanding, the influence of these essences heightens its impact, creating a look that is memorable, high-energy, and deeply expressive.

Jewel tones, icy brights, and crisp black-and-white contrasts remain flattering, but they are best expressed through bold styling choices, luxurious textures, and statement details that exude presence. Rather than soft draping or subtle blending, the Bold Winter thrives in rich, high-impact color pairings, striking silhouettes, and an overall sense of intensity, whether through dramatic lines or sumptuous, glamorous elements.

The G designation indicates an undercurrent of strong, yang energy within this blend. This adds an air of command

and presence, reinforcing the sharp contrasts and striking combinations that make Winter so bold. A Bold Winter G naturally carries the deepest, most saturated colors from the Winter palette and benefits from styling that leans into strong contrasts, edgy details, and an assertive, high-fashion aesthetic.

The T designation indicates a softer, more yin energy within this blend. This enhances the alluring, luxurious side of the Winter palette, creating a bold yet sensual and elegant effect. A Bold Winter T may favor plush fabrics, rich embellishments, and fluid shapes that maintain intensity without relying on strict structure, allowing for a powerful yet irresistibly captivating presence.

Playful Winter

The *Playful Winter* type combines the cool, high-contrast coloring of Winter with the youthful, small-scale nature of the Gamine and/or Ingenue style essences. While Winter's palette is typically bold and intense, the influence of these essences adds a sense of lightness, energy, and charm, creating a look that is striking yet approachable.

Icy pastels, crisp jewel tones, and bright contrasts remain flattering, but they are best expressed through smaller-scale patterns, tailored yet lively silhouettes, and playful styling elements that enhance their fresh and dynamic presence. Instead of long flowing lines or stark minimalism, the Playful Winter thrives in animated shapes, refined details, and an overall sense of youthful vibrancy, blending Winter's high contrast with a lively, eye-catching essence.

The G designation indicates an undercurrent of strong, yang energy within this blend. This adds a bold, spunky edge to the Playful Winter aesthetic, reinforcing the sharp contrast and structured styling often seen in Gamine influences. A Playful Winter G naturally carries vivid, high-contrast color combinations and benefits from crisp tailoring, bold accessories, and an energetic, expressive style that makes a statement.

The T designation indicates a softer, more yin energy within this blend. This enhances the delicate, whimsical side of the Winter palette, creating a look that is playful yet sweet and enchanting. A Playful Winter T may gravitate toward softer, icy hues and rounded details, favoring gentle textures, refined embellishments, and an overall sense of light, youthful elegance that maintains Winter's brightness in a more delicate way.

Classic Winter

The *Classic Winter* type combines the cool, high-contrast coloring of Winter with the timeless, balanced nature of the Classic essence. While Winter's palette is naturally bold and striking, the influence of Classic refines its intensity into a polished, harmonious aesthetic, creating a look that is sophisticated, structured, and effortlessly elegant.

Deep jewel tones, crisp whites, and rich blacks remain flattering, but they are best expressed through clean lines, symmetrical silhouettes, and high-quality fabrics that emphasize precision and refinement. Instead of exaggerated styling or extreme contrasts, the Classic Winter thrives in understated luxury, tailored fits, and an overall sense of poised confidence, blending Winter's depth with a balanced, timeless essence.

The G designation indicates an undercurrent of strong, yang energy within this blend. This adds a commanding presence and sharp definition to the Classic Winter aesthetic, reinforcing structured tailoring, sleek styling, and an air of quiet authority. A Classic Winter G naturally carries crisp, high-contrast color combinations and benefits from minimalist, well-tailored pieces and bold yet refined accessories that exude effortless power.

The T designation indicates a softer, more yin energy within this blend. This enhances the graceful, elegant side of the Winter palette, creating a look that is classic yet slightly softer and more approachable. A Classic Winter T may gravitate toward smoother textures, gently tailored pieces, and polished details, favoring graceful lines and a sophisticated, timeless charm that maintains Winter's cool contrast with a more refined ease.

The ColorEssence System bridges color analysis and personal style by recognizing that an individual's best colors must work in harmony with their natural movement, scale, and overall aesthetic presence. This approach ensures that people do not just wear colors that suit them, but also express their essence authentically and cohesively.

With 16 refined profiles, the ColorEssence System provides a customized, intuitive way to build a wardrobe that is not only flattering but deeply aligned with personal identity.

To learn more, visit **youniformbook.com**.

Appendix B: Youniform Activities

Throughout this book I have integrated activities and experiments to learn more about your style. I believe that personal style should belong to us, rather than having someone else tell us what to wear. Here you will find the comprehensive list of all included activities, organized by chapter, and a brief overview.

Chapter One

- Morning Decisions - make a list of your daily decision making and perform an analysis to see patterns.
- Tomorrow's Outfit Today - lay out your clothes for the day and wear them no matter what.
- Decide Who You Are - quick journaling activity to get clarity on who you want to be.

Chapter Two

- Cost per Wear Analysis - look at your recent purchases and decide their long-term value in your closet.

- Fashion Brand Research - discover the ethics of the companies where you buy clothes.
- Find Your Fibers - check your clothing to see what materials they are made of.

Chapter Three

- What Was She Wearing? - see if you can remember the details of a friend's outfit.
- Flaunt Your Favorite - put on your favorite item of clothing and spend time reflecting on why you love it.

Chapter Four

- Color Coded Closet - organize and arrange your entire closet by color.
- Style Goals Exercise - choose three conceptual words to frame your personal style.
- Body Silhouette Sketch - outline your body to become familiar with your shape.
- Closet Inventory - quick snapshot of what's currently in your closet.
- Style Affirmation - commit to the journey of exploring your personal style.

Chapter Five

- Picture Your Youniform - brainstorm your one perfect outfit.
- What's Your Magic Number - how many items do you think you need for the perfect wardrobe?
- Is it the One? - analyze your current outfit using the Youniform parameters.
- Get the Youniform Planner - visit **youniformbook.com** to get your planner and start creating your Youniforms.

Chapter Six

- Where to Wear? - analyze your outfit for the different areas of life it could fit.
- Lifestyle Audit - perform an audit of one average month to determine your Youniform needs.
- Workhorse or Wacky? - count your go to items and those that never work.

Chapter Seven

- Nature Color Study - look at various naturally occurring settings and images to see color cohesion.
- Attribute Assignment - discover your Big Four Season using hue, value, and chroma.

- Create a Color Palette - visit **youniformbook.com** to get your color palette template to design your closet.

Chapter Eight

- Brand Yourself - explore how you want to communicate your values through style as a personal brand.
- Essence Exploration - explore which essences are most dominant in your Essence Triad.

Chapter Nine

- Primary Accommodation - what is the singular physical aspect you need to consider when getting dressed?
- Clothing Style Analysis - use your newfound garment knowledge to assess your outfit.
- Body Neutrality Journaling - follow the prompts to make peace with your body.

Chapter Ten

- Master Shopping List - build your shopping list with top five items prioritized.
- Find Your Tags - evaluate your decluttering mindset by finding all your unworn new items.

Chapter Eleven

- Be Remembered - complete the legacy discovery statement.
- Reflect and Reach - complete the final assessment and email it to us at admin@radiantlydressed.com.

Recommended Reading

Below are many of the books I had read over the years related to personal style. Some of them I disagree with points, but all I found valuable to increasing my understanding of the intricacies of personal style.

Project 333 by Courtney Carver. The one that started it all for me; a true pioneer of minimalistic style.

Color Me a Season by Bernice Kentner. This is an undiscovered gem for color analysis, and one we require our Certification students to read as part of their curriculum.

Loved Clothes Last by Orsola de Castro. A great study on reframing clothes as assets instead of throwaway items.

The Power of Style by Bobbie Thomas. This had so many good practical nuggets for making style easier.

The Curated Closet by Anuschka Rees. A personal favorite that taught me so many things early in my journey.

Beyond Beautiful by Anuschka Rees. I binged this one after the previous and it was revelatory on self image.

Overdressed by Elizabeth L. Cline. This book has so many nuggets about the fashion industry and what is wrong.

Lessons from Madame Chic by Jennifer L. Scott. This one was so fun for learning about the French approach to fashion and style.

Fashionopolis by Dana Thomas. This is a really heavy read on every intricate part of the fashion industry.

Let it Go by Peter Walsh. A stark look at not holding on to things just because and a new mindset to stop collecting.

David Kibbe's Power of Style. An updated look at the full Kibbe Style Identity system.

References

Addad. 2022. "How Linen Fabric Is Made: In-Depth Guide." Son de Flor. January 27, 2022. https://sondeflor.com/blogs/all-about-linen/how-linen-fabric-is-made?srsltid=AfmBOorabecPDnisKCpE5R1qX3dFkH3W0gMpLi1zWCojW5vRrxgmzecT.

Brown, Amy. 2023. "Resale Is All the Rage, but Fashion Brands Not Making a Dent in Unsustainable Levels of Waste." *Reuters*, August 9, 2023, sec. Climate & Energy. https://www.reuters.com/sustainability/climate-energy/resale-is-all-rage-fashion-brands-not-making-dent-unsustainable-levels-waste-2023-08-09/.

Burleigh, Emma. 2025. "Gen Alpha Is Snubbing the Careers That Boomers Dreamed Of. As Influencers Become the New Faces of Entrepreneurship, They Want In." Fortune. April 26, 2025. https://fortune.com/article/gen-alpha-dream-careers-youtuber-influencer-social-media/.

Cardona, Nancy. 2025. "Global Apparel Industry Statistics (2024) | UniformMarket." Uniform Market. 2025.

https://www.uniformmarket.com/statistics/global-apparel-industry-statistics.

Carnegie, Dale. 1936. How to Win Friends and Influence People. London: Vermilion.

Clean Clothes Campaign. 2015. "Who Paid up and Who Failed to Take Responsibility?" Clean Clothes Campaign. 2015. https://cleanclothes.org/campaigns/past/rana-plaza/who-paid-up-and-who-failed-to-take-responsibility.

Dabir, Sam. 2024. "The Neuroscience of Decision Making." Uwo.ca. 2024. https://uwo.ca/se/thrive/blog/2024/the-neuroscience-of-decision-making.html.j

Edwards, Scott. 2016. "Sugar and the Brain." Hms.harvard.edu. Harvard Medical School. 2016. https://hms.harvard.edu/news-events/publications-archive/brain/sugar-brain.

Edwards, Sharon. 2024. "How the 'Father of Haute Couture' Revolutionised Fashion." *BBC*, December 26, 2024. https://www.bbc.com/news/articles/ckg7l2j43l4o.

Gallo, Carmine. "Steve Jobs' Surprise IPhone Reveal Is Still A Presentation Classic." Forbes. Forbes Media LLC, June 30, 2022. https://www.forbes.com/sites/carminegallo/2022/06/30/steve-jobs-surprise-iphone-reveal-is-still-a-presentation-classic/.

Galloway, Kathryn . 2024. "The Environmental Impact of Cotton Production." International Science Council. June 17, 2024. https://council.science/blog/the-environmental-impact-of-cotton-production/.

Gillebaart, Marleen. 2018. "The 'Operational' Definition of Self-Control." *Frontiers in Psychology* 9 (1231). https://doi.org/10.3389/fpsyg.2018.01231.

Helm, Mykhail. 2024. "Beneath the Seams: The Human Toll of Fast Fashion." Earth Day. September 9, 2024. https://www.earthday.org/beneath-the-seams-the-human-toll-of-fast-fashion/.

Hoskins, Tansy. 2014. "Luxury Brands: Higher Standards or Just a Higher Mark-Up?" The Guardian. The Guardian. December 10, 2014. https://www.theguardian.com/sustainable-business/2014/dec/10/luxury-brands-behind-gloss-same-dirt-ethics-production.

Igini, Martina. 2023. "10 Concerning Fast Fashion Waste Statistics." Earth.org. August 21, 2023. https://earth.org/statistics-about-fast-fashion-waste/.

James, L. (2022, July 27). *Mountains of clothes washed up on Ghana beach show cost of fast fashion.* The Independent. https://www.independent.co.uk/climate-change/news/fast-fashion-ghana-clothes-waste-b2132399.html

Kavishe, Ed. *Carolina Herrera*. Fashion Wire Press. Creative Commons Attribution–ShareAlike 3.0. https://commons.wikimedia.org/w/index.php?curid=412420 5

Kennemer, James. 2025. "Cosmo Sourcing." Cosmo Sourcing. February 3, 2025. https://www.cosmosourcing.com/blog/the-top-12-countries-for-clothing-garment-and-apparel-manufacturing.

Klerk, Amy de. 2016. "Women Spend 17 Minutes Each Morning Choosing an Outfit." Harper's BAZAAR. June 6, 2016. https://www.harpersbazaar.com/uk/people-parties/bazaar-at-work/news/a37318/women-average-time-choosing-outfit/.

Langley, Edward, Stefan Durkacz, and Simona Tanase. Rep. *Clothing Longevity and Measuring Active Use*. Waste and Resources Action Programme (WRAP), August 2013. https://www.wrap.ngo/sites/default/files/2021-04/Clothing %20Longevity%20Report.pdf?_gl=1*5xnnrg*_ga*MTkyOT QxOTU5OS4xNzQzNTA2MjUx*_ga_C43RKFPDL6*MTc 0MzUwNjI1MS4xLjAuMTc0MzUwNjI1MS4wLjAuMA.

Merriam Webster. 2025. "Definition of Communication." Merriam-Webster. 2025. https://www.merriam-webster.com/dictionary/communicati on.

McKnight, Rebecca. 2013. "A Woman's Outfit: 35% Weather, 14% Plans for the Day and 7% Mood - Her.ie." HER. October 10, 2013. https://her.ie/style/a-womans-outfit-35-weather-14-plans-for-the-day-and-7-mood-65278?cacheTtl=5&cacheKey=request-browser-httpswwwheriestylea-womans-outfit-35-weather-14-plans-for-the-day-and-7-mood65278.

New American Standard Bible. 1995. Nashville: Holman Bible Publishers.

"The Newborn Senses: Sight and Eye Color." n.d. Charlotte Lozier Institute.https://lozierinstitute.org/dive-deeper/the-newborn-senses-sight-and-eye-color/.

Nihart, Alexander J., Marcus A. Garcia, Eliane El Hayek, Rui Liu, Marian Olewine, Josiah D. Kingston, Eliseo F. Castillo, et al. 2025. "Bioaccumulation of Microplastics in Decedent Human Brains." Nature Medicine 31 (31). https://doi.org/10.1038/s41591-024-03453-1.

Nizzoli, Giada. 2024. "Brief History of Fast Fashion (& Changing Its Future Course) | Sustainable Fashion Blog| Project Cece." Www.projectcece.com. Project CeCe. April 10, 2024. https://www.projectcece.com/blog/637/brief-history-of-fast-fashion/.

Pantone. 2026. Pantone. 2026. https://www.pantone.com/articles/color-fundamentals/how-do-we-see-color?srsltid=AfmBOopvXrteCDXFzPX9TyqsTqgDXl71ayDw9CquWJNER7dO4YdXrTfN.

Raposo, Jacqueline . 2024. "What Is Spoon Theory Used For, and What Are Its Benefits?" GoodRx. June 7, 2024.

https://www.goodrx.com/health-topic/mental-health/spoon-theory.

"Scuba Diving Deaths per Year | Statistics and Causes." n.d. Www.private-Scuba.com. https://www.private-scuba.com/diving/injuries/death-statistics.html.

Stefanie. 2019. "History of the Sewing Machine: A Story Stitched in Scandal." Contrado Blog. June 26, 2019. https://www.contrado.com/blog/history-of-the-sewing-machine/?srsltid=AfmBOorjDDEzR6zfAGSc4jTMFuAohdRE4m8ywwYG49OQ8eaJEItbEZeJ.

Tonti, Lucianne. 2025. "Dirty Laundry: What Really Happens to Your Clothes When You Donate Them to Charity?" The Guardian. The Guardian. April 4, 2025. https://www.theguardian.com/australia-news/2025/apr/05/dirty-laundry-what-really-happens-to-your-clothes-when-you-donate-them-to-charity.

"US Home Organizers and Storage Market Size & Share Analysis - Industry Research Report - Growth Trends." n.d. Www.mordorintelligence.com. https://www.mordorintelligence.com/industry-reports/united-states-home-organizers-and-storage-market.

Valenzuela, Sebastián, Daniel Halpern, and James E. Katz. 2014. "Social Network Sites, Marriage Well-Being and Divorce: Survey and State-Level Evidence from the United States." *Computers in Human Behavior* 36 (July): 94–101. https://doi.org/10.1016/j.chb.2014.03.034.

Van der Weel, Ruud, and Audrey Van der Meer. 2024. “Handwriting but Not Typewriting Leads to Widespread Brain Connectivity: A High-Density EEG Study with Implications for the Classroom.” *Frontiers in Psychology* 14 (14). https://doi.org/10.3389/fpsyg.2023.1219945.

Woodtli, Thomas. *Sahara Desert.* Flickr. Creative Commons Attribution–ShareAlike 2.0. https://commons.wikimedia.org/w/index.php?curid=106548897

XAP Corporation. 2024. “RUReadyND - Article.” Nd.gov. 2024. https://secure.ruready.nd.gov/Home/Article.aspx?articleId=TKZjBonzsuebU8XAP2BPAXEAiXAP2FPAX11wXAP3DPAXXAP3DPAX&level=3XAP2FPAX6J7I3kztATGuYyXAP2BPAXDahIQXAP3DPAXXAP3DPAX

About the Author

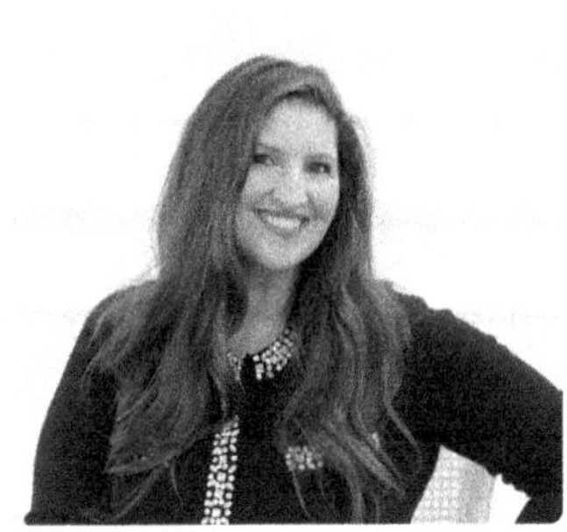

Stacey Herndon is an international style expert, color analyst, and educator whose work sits at the intersection of beauty, simplicity, and purpose. She is a member of the Association of Image Consultants International and the founder of Radiantly Dressed, a style education company that has reached more than 500,000 women and served more than 2,700 clients through courses, programs, and personalized style work.

Stacey is the creator of the Youniform Framework, a practical system designed to simplify how women get dressed without sacrificing beauty or intention. Her work grew out of years of observing patterns in how women think, decide, and feel about their clothes. Her neurodivergent brain has shaped her ability to see systems and to build frameworks that bring clarity, consistency, and relief to everyday decisions.

Her approach to style is grounded in a simple belief: beauty and simplicity are not opposites. Clothing is not the point, but it matters because it supports the life being lived. When style is aligned, it frees women to focus their energy on work, relationships, and callings that carry real weight and meaning.

In addition to her work with consumers, Stacey trains and certifies professional stylists through her ColorEssence program, where she teaches a structured, client-centered approach to color and style analysis rooted in discernment rather than rules.

A seventh-generation Texan, Stacey lives outside Houston with her husband and seven children. Despite the busy mornings, she gets dressed looking her best every day in under five minutes. Her mission is to help women show up with intention, authenticity, and the confidence to live a bold and radiant life.

Let's Connect

YOUNIFORMBOOK.COM

I would love to welcome you into our Radiant World and help you build a wardrobe that lets you live a meaningful life. Here are several ways to connect with me:

1. Your book purchase includes complimentary access to our private reader support group. Visit **youniformbook.com** and complete the form to receive your invitation. Inside, you'll find additional resources, conversation, and guidance to help you apply what you've learned.

2. If you want to keep learning, visit **radiantlydressed.com** for over 100 in-depth articles on personal style, color, wardrobe planning, and getting dressed with intention. This is a free resource designed to support you wherever you are.

3. I regularly share insights, behind-the-scenes moments, and practical style guidance across our platforms:
   Instagram: instagram.com/radiantlydressed
   Facebook: facebook.com/radiantlydressed
   LinkedIn: linkedin.com/in/stacey-herndon/
   YouTube: youtube.com/@staceyherndon
   Substack: staceyherndon.substack.com/

4. If you prefer to work at your own pace, visit **radiantstyleshop.com** to explore nearly 100 self-guided products covering color, wardrobe planning, outfit creation, and many of the concepts introduced in this book.

5. If you want support, accountability, and access to me as your stylist, our group coaching program offers a full style curriculum that expands on the book, along with individualized feedback. Learn more and apply at **iamaradiantwoman.com**.

6. If this book sparked interest in turning style into meaningful work, learn more about our professional training and certification programs at **coloressencestylesystem.com**.

7. For workshops, retreats, conferences, special events, or custom collaborations, visit **staceyherndon.com** to connect.

www.ingramcontent.com/pod-product-compliance
Ingram Content Group UK Ltd.
Pitfield, Milton Keynes, MK11 3LW, UK
UKHW021926300326
11591UKWH00004B/526

9 798994 154229